THE GULF WAR
AND
MENTAL HEALTH

THE GULF WAR
——AND——
MENTAL HEALTH

A Comprehensive Guide

Edited by
JAMES A. MARTIN,
LINETTE R. SPARACINO,
and GREGORY BELENKY

PRAEGER

Westport, Connecticut
London

Library of Congress Cataloging-in-Publication Data

The Gulf War and mental health : a comprehensive guide / edited by
   James A. Martin, Linette R. Sparacino, and Gregory Belenky.
      p.   cm.
   Includes bibliographical references (p.   ) and index.
   ISBN 0–275–95631–8 (alk. paper)
      1. Persian Gulf War, 1991—Psychological aspects.   2. War
   neuroses.   3. Military psychiatry.   I. Martin, James A. (James
   Ashworth).   II. Sparacino, Linette R.   III. Belenky,
   Gregory.
   DS79.744.P78G85   1996
   956.7044′2—dc20   96–2200

British Library Cataloguing in Publication Data is available.

Library of Congress Catalog Card Number: 96–2200
ISBN: 0–275–95631–8

First published in 1996

Praeger Publishers, 88 Post Road West, Westport, CT 06881
An imprint of Greenwood Publishing Group, Inc.

Printed in the United States of America

The paper used in this book complies with the
Permanent Paper Standard issued by the National
Information Standards Organization (Z39.48–1984).

10 9 8 7 6 5 4 3 2 1

Contents

Foreword

Robert T. Joy

This book deals with the acute and chronic behavioral responses to battle. The chapters assume the conventional definitions of stress and *posttraumatic stress disorder* (PTSD) and take us through the behavioral science and military medical preparations for the Persian Gulf War. As is usual in the U.S. Army, we are never quite prepared to go to war, and in 1990, the Army Medical Department shared in that unreadiness (GAO, 1992). The operational working out of providing preventive and therapeutic psychiatric care for combat stress is the real theme of this book.

It is the nomenclature of the conditions described that I wish to discuss. Absent a specific etiology, medicine uses words such as condition and syndrome. Psychiatrists characterize a disorder in terms of the patient's words, behavior, and past history as defined by the current psychiatric assumptions about behavioral dysfunction. In common with much of medicine (and life), we believe that naming something means that we understand it, at least in part. But that naming often has an unappreciated long history. Rosenberg (1988), our best social historian of medicine, introduced the idea of "framing" disease (which has been further applied by Cunningham [1992]).

Disease is at once a biological event, a generation specific repertoire of verbal constructs reflecting medicine's intellectual and institutional history; potential legitimization for public policy; an aspect of social role and individual intrapsychic identity; a sanction for cultural values and a structuring element in doctor and patient interactions. In some ways disease does not exist until we have agreed that it does, by perceiving, naming and responding to it. (Rosenberg, 1988, xiii–xxvi)

It is this conceptualization that I shall follow in this foreword.

I begin examination of the diagnostic labels with stress. Its use in modern terms dates back to 1303, according to the Oxford English Dictionary. The introduction of and popularization of stress in modern medicine may fairly be attributed to Hans Selye, who limited the response to stress to the endocrine system and said nothing about behavioral responses (Selye, 1936; 1946). The Oxford English Dictionary also documents that neurosis is an old word; in varying usages it dates from 1797, but in modern terms it appears to have entered medicine in 1874 and was common by 1896. It is important to recognize that the *etiology* and *clinical definition* of neurosis varied according to the medical and cultural theories of any given period. Finally, shock in the sense of a disturbed behavior due to "an unwelcome occurrence" dates back to 1705 and as "nervous exhaustion" to 1804.

A post-battle behavioral "disorder" has been suggested in the U.S. Civil War "nostalgia," which is a retrospective diagnosis thoroughly destroyed by Rosen (1975). It has been suggested that the present-day views of a sudden traumatic incident lending to acute and chronic symptoms identical to those discussed in this book began in the 1860s as "railway spine" (Caplan, 1995). Initially considered a post-accident concussive injury with neurological damage, it soon became defined as a psychic disorder, variously neuromimesis, traumatic hysteria, or neurasthenia. Secondary gain from suits against the railroad company and medicolegal arguments from both sides clouded the issue, but by the 1890s, rest and "suggestion by the doctor" were the preferred treatment. A neurosurgeon, while not disagreeing with the psychiatric component, has suggested that vertebral compression fracture could have been responsible for some of the symptoms (Keller, 1995).

The Russo-Japanese War of 1904–1905 may mark the first application of formal psychiatric care to patients with "psychoses" variously recorded as hysterical, neurasthenic, and manic-depressive with the etiology and clinical descriptions appearing to approximate modern combat stress (Richards, 1910). World War I saw behavioral dysfunction that was initially defined as cowardice, desertion, malingering, "wandering away," and "losing their heads," but it was soon recognized that brave soldiers could have these symptoms. "Stress" (in the environmental sense, in this case battle) was considered the precipitating cause of "war neurosis" in "constitutionally inferior individuals" (Salmon, 1929).

Was this then an illness? Diagnoses such as hysteria, neurasthenia, and traumatic psychoneurosis began to appear as early as 1914. Shellshock— initially believed to be the etiology of this constellation of symptoms by traumatic overpressure—as a *word* may have been invented by a noncommissioned officer (Ritchie, 1986). It is not my purpose to examine the history of shellshock; that is done in many reviews; for a recent excellent discussion see Merskey (1991). Shellshock became both the lay term and generally the medical one. *Etiology* at the pathophysiological level was referred to as either predisposition or nervous tendency or to the various hypotheses proposed by the increasingly influential psychoanalytical theories of Freud (1918).

Framing World War I shellshock in the British Army in Rosenberg's terms has been carefully done by Ritchie (1986, pp 247 252) and Feudtner, from slightly different perspectives (Feudtner, 1993). They argue that the brutality of trench warfare was the social and cultural context in which "transient paraplegia from shell explosions" and "hysterical and neurasthenic breakdowns" could occur. The physiological and behavioral responses represented various combinations of physical injury, hereditary predisposition, "nervous and mental exhaustion," and the working out of neuroses. It is not the purpose of this forward to extend this discussion into the issues of selection of therapies; "macronegotiation" of the disease between soldier and medical officer; the interactions between line and medical officers about shellshock; and so on. The reader is referred to the work of Ritchie (1986), Merskey (1991), and Feudtner (1993) for thorough, insightful discussion.

When World War II arrived for the United States in 1941, preparation for the care of shellshock cases was absent (Strecker and Appel, 1945; Hausman and Rioch, 1967). While the lessons of World War I were being relearned, the term shellshock had been replaced by anxiety neurosis, acute anxiety states, and psychogenic disturbances. These words, implying some sort of mental disease or psychiatric breakdown, were both unintelligible and unacceptable to line officers. These diagnostic statements led to pentothal abreaction treatment, evacuation of patients to rear area hospitals (never to return to the front), and an unacceptable manpower drain from combat units (Grinker and Spiegel, 1943). Captain Frederick R. Hanson, (Medical Corps, U.S. Army), a neurologist, had served with Canadian and British troops before the United States entered the war. He was familiar with British studies of *battle neurosis* or *not yet diagnosed (nervous)*. The British eventually settled on the term *battle exhaustion* or *exhaustion*. In early 1942, the British Consultant in Psychiatry, Brigadier G. W. B. James, introduced the term *exhaustion* and *campaign neuroses* in the Eighth Army in North Africa (Copp and McAndrew, 1990).

Exhaustion had no implications of mental disease and was an acceptable diagnosis to line commanders. The etiology was the stress of battle and a general social acceptance that everyone has his breaking point. Major General Omar Bradley's directive of April 26th, 1943 on holding policy ratified the word, which now became the diagnosis as a matter of policy (Glass, 1973). Interestingly, Lieutenant General Robert L. Eichelberger, commanding the medically disastrous 1942 Buna battle in New Guinea, noted that "I had seen men lying in ditches, weeping with battle shock." This is the first use of the term I have found (Eichelberger, 1950). Of course, not all senior commanders accepted the term exhaustion. To Lieutenant General George S. Patton, Jr., it was simply cowardice. D'Este argued that Patton had combat exhaustion when he slapped two patients in notorious incidents (D'Este, 1995).

Combat fatigue appears to have been the preferred term in the Pacific Theater, but the etiological and social assumptions were those of the European Theater (Glass, 1973, p. 594). *Combat exhaustion* or *fatigue* had completely replaced all uses of any psychiatric terms, and *neurosis* had disappeared from the diagnostic nosology. *Immaturity reactions* now named those soldiers previously called psychoneurotic due to predisposing factors (Glass, 1973, pp. 992–994).

The social and medical acceptance of *breaking point* now meant that the stress (combat) could overwhelm *anyone*; that it was a normal behavior and that acknowledging and accepting fear was a part of being in combat. That was the U.S. Army position.

The Royal Air Force (RAF) and the U.S. Army Air Force held different views. The RAF—culturally defining courage by class and character (both a function of the upper end of the social scale)—used the terms *lack of moral fiber*, *lack of confidence*, and *fear of flying* early in a combat tour. Such patients were handled administratively. This appears to be a residue of a British response to shellshock in World War I (Bogacz, 1989). On the other hand, those who had performed well in extended combat and "broke" were labeled medically as "anxiety state." The U.S. Army Air Force, lacking a social class determinant, used the terms *temperamentally unsuitable* and *psychological failure* as lack-of-moral-fiber equivalents. Such aircrew were—as in the RAF —disposed of administratively. Those who had endured were considered to be medical patients and were classified as *flying fatigue*, *operational fatigue* or *exhaustion* or *fear reaction*. Early in the war (1942–1943), the diagnoses of airmen were *anxiety reaction* and *psychoneurosis*—this led to Grinker's pentothal abreaction therapy discussed earlier. For a magisterial treatment of cross-cultural understanding and management of combat stress reaction, see Wells (1995).

Interesting cross-cultural studies introduce a larger language. In World War II, the German army used *stress breakdown*, *war hysterics* or *neurosis*, and a symptom that named the condition—*scheuttelsz* (trembler) (Schneider, 1987). Field orders of the German army in Sicily in 1943 required "rigid discipline," e.g., cooperate or be shot. "Examples of individuals always work wonders," and soldiers exhibiting "signs of indiscipline or panic were to be clubbed or shot" (D'Este, 1991). The Australian army in World War II apparently clung to neurotic etiologies for war neurosis, anxiety state, battle strain or combat stress or exhaustion (terms essentially interchangeable). Interestingly, it is twice noted that female nurses are immune, even when stressed (Walker, 1952).

As acute behavioral maladaption began to be a problem in the Israeli Defense Force in the 1970s, they used "combat reaction" with acute and chronic manifestations. The Israelis were willing to consider personality predisposition a factor in chronic PTSD (Noy, 1987).

The diagnostic categories appear to have changed between World Wars I and II (from conversion hysteria to psychosomatic disorders); this is clearly a reflection of changing medical theory and nosology interacting with a social vocabulary (Neill, 1993). American psychiatry, influenced in part by the outpatient management of combat exhaustion, changed its professional focus from the inpatient asylum to outpatient community psychiatry and its therapeutic attention from the psychoses to the neuroses (Grob, 1987, 1990). The new psychodynamic psychiatry is clearly reflected in the Army Medical Department consultant committee of 1946, which urged legitimization of the term *combat exhaustion* (Bartemeier et al., 1946). The decreasing emphasis on biological causes for behavioral dysfunction; the enlarging concepts of environment–mind interactions; an enhanced use of community mental health programs; and governmental, educational, and insurance requirements for a new and "epidemiologically useful" nosology led to the publication of the first *Diagnostic and Statistical Manual* (DSM I) by the American Psychiatric Association in 1952. As the new nomenclature was taught and used, the etiological definitions of mental illness were shaped by psychodynamic and psychoanalytic assumptions (Grob, 1991).

Thus combat exhaustion, with all the assumptions about normal behavior, breaking points, stress and the normality of fear in battle, became fixed in etiology and nomenclature in Korea (Hausman and Rioch, 1967) and Vietnam (Bourne, 1976).

Finally, Belenky has described the disorder as an expanded "combat reaction spectrum," from immediate (combat reaction, battle shock, shell shock, and explosion blow), through acute (combat fatigue, battle fatigue, and acute posttraumatic stress disorder), through delayed (reactions during combat lulls, while home on pass, following rapid demobilization), though late (old sergeant syndrome, delayed PTSD), and, finally, chronic reactions (war neurosis and chronic PTSD). This is exclusively an environmental etiology nosology and does not assume either biological or predisposing factors, except possibly in the chronic states (Belenky, 1987).

The United States has paid some attention to psychiatric illness in veterans, with a tentative interest after World War I, although most attention was paid to discharged psychotics (Williams, 1929). After World War II, attention was paid to reintegration of the veteran to civil life (Brill and Kupper, 1966). There soon were reports of residual effects of combat. The Veteran's Administration evaluated 1475 men who had been hospitalized for psychoneurosis in 1944; 25 percent had moderate to severe psychosomatic complaints (Brill and Beebe, 1955). Other authors predicted that the symptoms after combat exhaustion could persist and that they could be delayed or chronic (Grinker and Spiegel, 1945; Kardiner, 1947).

However, it was the Vietnam War, plagued by political quarrels, lack of home support, drug abuse, and perceived defeat, that led to general public recognition of PTSD and changes in social policy and medical nomenclature (Shatan, 1973; Haley, 1974; Egendorf et al., 1981). However, the formal psychiatric nosology had changed. In DSM I (1952), the World War II experience led to the introduction of gross stress reaction, not a neurosis and temporary in duration. But DSM II (1968) dropped this term and made no obvious substitution.

However, psychiatrists and social workers treating Vietnam veterans in VA hospitals and an organized group of antiwar Vietnam veterans led a political, social, and medical movement for recognition of PTSD and negotiated with American Psychiatric Association leaders from 1974 to 1978 in a biopolitical struggle that eventually introduced PTSD as an accepted term in DSM III (1980) (Scott, 1990).

So we have seen the name of a behavior change as the social context changed. A neurosis due to trauma in civil life was variously termed malingering (to be punished) or cowardice (which could get one shot) in the military. In World War I, medical officers initially sought a traumatic etiology for shellshock. When that failed, the behavior was either preconditioned as constitutional and neurotic or class specific and derived from some personal failure such as lack of character or being a weakling. The failure of these models in World War II led to exhaustion or fatigue—both tied to battle or combat with the behavior defined as an environmental challenge that could affect everyone. This nosology pleased nearly all combat arms commanders because it avoided the stigmata of mental illness.

I thus argue that combat stress reaction, a behavior caused by a particular environment in a special place and time, has been so named today because it presently satisfies Rosenberg's (1988) criteria for disease. All his variables have interacted variously over time—the social, political, medical, cultural (military), and, at some level, biological—as determinants that allow us to identify a particular cluster of behaviors. We are comfortable with what has been wrought and we have conditioned our combat commanders that fear is normal, that they can and should thus indoctrinate their soldiers, do preventive therapy and demand posttraumatic intervention from psychiatrists (Fontenot, 1995). These ideas would horrify a line commander in 1910.

It is possibly cynical to suggest that poets may have a clearer vision than we do of the power of words. Consider Carroll's *Through the Looking Glass* (Chapter 6) that includes the following passage:

"When *I* use a word," Humpty Dumpty said, in rather a scornful tone, "it means just what I choose it to mean neither more nor less." "The question is," said Alice, "whether you *can* make words mean so many different things." "The question is," said Humpty Dumpty, "which is to be master—that's all."

If Humpty Dumpty is right, what meaning has "combat stress reaction?" Are there "accident stress reactions," or "mugging stress reactions" and so on? Stress has been so conflated that it can mean almost anything. And if reaction is a maladaption—is combat stress action to be taken as heroism or the enjoyment of combat?

I prefer Shakespeare's lines (*Hamlet, III*, 2, 20) because they urge a sense of caution: "Suit the action to the word, the word to the action; with this special observance, that you o'erstep not the modesty of nature." We need to remember that modesty in the context of combat stress reaction when our successors better frame the nature of the condition with an even deeper understanding of the behavior they are observing.

REFERENCES

Bartemeier, L., L. Kubie, W. Menninger, .J. Romano, and J. D. Whitehorn. (1946). "Combat exhaustion." *J. Nerv. Ment. Dis.*, 104:358–359, 489–525.

Belenky, G. L. (1987). "Varieties of reaction and adaption to combat experience." *Bull. Menninger Clinic*, 51:64–79.

Bogacz, T. (1989). "War neurosis and cultural change in England, 1914–1922: The work of the War Office Committee of Enquiry into shellshock." *J. Contemp. Hist.*, 24:227–256.

Bourne, P. G. (1976). *Men, Stress and Vietnam*. Boston: Little, Brown and Co., 8–9.

Brill, N. Q. and G. W. Beebe. (1955). "A Follow-up Study of War Neurosis." *VA Medical Monograph Series*. Washington, D.C.: USGPO.

Brill, N. Q. and H. I. Kupper. (1966). "Problems of adjustment in return to civilian life." In A. J. Glass and R. J. Bernucci (eds.), *Medical Department, United States Army, Neuropsychiatry in World War II*, Vol. I. Washington, D.C.: OTSG, USGPO, 721–727.

Caplan, E. (1995). "Trains, brains, and sprains: Railway spine and the origins of psychoneurosis." *Bull. Hist. Med.*, 69:387–419.

Copp, T. and B. McAndrew. (1990). *Battle Exhaustion: Soldiers and Psychiatrists in the Canadian Army, 1939–1945*. Montreal: McGill-Queen's University Press, 22–25, 44–50.

Cunningham, A. (1992). "Transforming plague: The laboratory and the identity of infectious disease." In A. Cunningham and P. Williams (eds.), *The Laboratory Revolution in Medicine*. Cambridge: Cambridge University Press, 209–244.

D'Este, C. (1991). *Bitter Victory*. New York: Harper, 495–496.

D'Este, C. (1995). *Patton: A Genius for War*. New York: HarperCollins, 533–546.

Egendorf, A., C. Kadushin, R. S. Lauter, G. Rothbart, and L. Sloan. (1981). *Legacies of Vietnam: Comparative Adjustment of Veterans and Their Peers*. Washington, D.C.: USGPO.

Eichelberger, R. L. (1950). *Our Jungle Road to Tokyo*. New York: Doubleday, 69.

Feudtner, C. (1993). "Minds the dead have ravished: Shellshock, history and the ecology of disease systems." *Hist. Sci.*, 31:377–420.

Fontenot, G. (1995). "Fear God and Dreadnought." *Mil. Review*, 75:13–24.

Freud, S. (1918). *Reflections on War and Death*. New York: Moffatt.

Glass, A. J. (ed.), (1973). *Medical Department, United States Army, Neuropsychiatry in World War II*, Vol. II. Washington, D.C.: OTSG, USGPO, 6–12.

Government Accounting Office (GAO). (August 1992). *Operation Desert Storm: Full Army Medical Capability Not Achieved*, GAO Report NSIAD-92-175.

Grinker, R. R. and J. P. Spiegel. (1943). *War Neuroses in North Africa: The Tunisian Campaign*. New York: Josiah Macy Foundation.

Grinker, R. R. and J. P. Spiegel. (1945). *Men Under Stress*. Philadelphia: Blakiston.

Grob, G. N. (1987). "The forging of mental health policy in America: World War II to New Frontier." *J. Hist. Med. Allied Sci.*, 42:410–446.

Grob, G. N. (1990). "World War II and American psychiatry." *Psychohist. Rev.*, 19:41–69.

Grob, G. N. (1991). "Origins of DSM-I: A study in appearance and reality." *Amer. J. Psychiatry*, 148:421–431.

Haley, S. A. (1974). "When the patient reports atrocities: Specific treatment considerations of the Vietnam Veteran." *Arch. Gen. Psychiatry*, 30:191–196.

Hausman, H. and D. McK. Rioch. (1967). "Military psychiatry." *Arch. Gen. Psych.*, 16:727–739.

Kardiner, A. (1947). *War, Stress and Neurotic Illness*. New York: Hoeber.

Keller, T. (1995). "Railway spine revisited: Traumatic neurosis or neurotrauma?" *J. Hist. Med. Allied Sci.*, 50:507–524.

Merskey, H. (1991). "Shellshock." In G. E. Berrios and H. Freeman (eds.), *150 Years of British Psychiatry, 1841–1991*. London: Gaskell, 245–267.

Neill, J. R. (1993). "How psychiatric symptoms varied in World War I and II." *Mil. Med.*, 158:149–151.

Noy, S. (1987). "Stress and personality as factors in the causation and prognosis of combat reaction." In G. Belenky (ed.), *Contemporary Studies in Combat Psychiatry*. New York: Greenwood, 20–29.

Richards, R. L. (1910). "Mental and nervous diseases in the Russo-Japanese War." *Mil. Surgeon*, 26:177–193.

Ritchie, R. D. (1986). *One History of Shellshock*. Ph.D. dissertation. San Diego: University of California (University Microfilm 8622880).

Rosen, G. (1975). "Nostalgia. A forgotten psychological disorder." *Psychol. Med.*, 5:340–354.

Rosenberg, C. E. (1988). "Introduction. Framing disease: Illness, society and history." In C. E. Rosenberg and J. Golden (eds.), *Framing Disease, Studies in Cultural History*. New Brunswick, N.J.: Rutgers University Press, xiii–xxvi.

Salmon, T. (1929). "Introduction." In P. Bailey, F. E. Williams and P. O. Komora (eds.), *Medical Department of the United States Army in the World War, Vol. X, Neuropsychiatry*. Washington, D.C.: USGPO, 1–3.

Schneider, R. J. (1987). "Stress breakdown in the Wehrmacht: Implications for today's army." In G. Belenky (ed.), *Contemporary Studies in Combat Psychiatry*. New York: Greenwood, 87–101.

Scott, W. J. (1990). "PTSD in DSM-III: A case in the politics of diagnosis and disease." *Social Problems*, 37:294–310.

Selye, H. (1936). "A syndrome produced by diverse nocuous agents." *Nature*, 138:32.

Selye, H. (1946). "The general adaption syndrome and the diseases of adaption." *J. Clin. Endocrin.*, 6:117–200.

Shatan, C. F. (1973). "The grief of soldiers in mourning: Vietnam combat veterans' self help movement." *Amer. J. Orthopsych.*, 43:640–653.

Strecker, E. A. and K. E. Appel. (1945). *Psychiatry in Modern Warfare*. New York: Macmillan, 5–7.

Walker, A. S. (1952). *Australia in the War of 1939–1945, Medical Series, Vol. I, Clinical Problems of War*. Canberra: Australian War Memorial, 674–707.

Wells, M. K. (1995). *Courage and Air Warfare: The Allied Aircrew Experience in the Second World War*. London: Frank Cass, 161–208.

Williams, F. E. (1929). "Disposition of mental cases." In P. Bailey, F. Williams, and P. Komora (eds.), *The Medical Department of the United States Army in the World War. Vol. X, Neuropsychiatry*. Washington, D.C.: USGPO, 139–149.

Preface

Faris R. Kirkland

Twenty years ago, the United States Army began a process of continuous renovation (Dunnigan and Macedonia, 1993; Kittfield, 1995; Meyer and Ancel, 1995). The rapid and dramatic evolution in doctrine, training, and equipment arising from this process has received deserved praise following the dramatic victory in the Persian Gulf War. Less obvious but more radical and difficult to achieve have been changes in the human dimensions of the Army arising from growing understanding of the extent to which psychological and social processes affect combat readiness. The key to reform in the human dimensions has been a growing trust and respect between the leaders of line units and members of the military mental health community. Three of the chapters in this book—those by Holsenbeck, Campbell and Engel, and Sutton and Clark—provide concrete examples.

For more than a century, the Army has considered the emotional well being of the soldier under three rubrics: morale, spiritual concerns, and psychiatric breakdown. Commanders are responsible for, and dependent for their success in combat on, morale. Morale is the set of perceptions soldiers have about their prospects for success and survival and the virtue of their cause. It is the product of the troops' belief in their own and their leaders' competence, the success of commanders in providing for their troops' welfare, and the combat environment.

Chaplains (or priests, in the early centuries of recorded history) have provided warriors with spiritual support. The modern military chaplaincy assists soldiers in reconciling the behavior necessary in war with their moral values, and helps them deal with deaths of comrades and their own possible deaths.

Robert T. Joy, in his foreword, describes how interactions among the values and perspectives of military psychiatrists, soldiers, and the public have led to halting but progressive understanding of psychological breakdown in combat. The period of most dramatic expansion in awareness and management of combat stress has occurred in the past decade. James Stokes explains in his chapter how the Persian Gulf War caught the Army in the midst of major changes in doctrine and organization for combat stress control.

COMMAND AND MEDICAL ACTION IN THE HUMAN DIMENSIONS

Although Army Regulations have stated the principles of leadership that produce high morale since the early part of the nineteenth century, implementation of those principles has been the exception rather than the rule (Kirkland, 1990). Among the lessons from the war in Vietnam was recognition that rapid turnover of personnel, poor communication across ranks, and discrepant perceptions and goals among soldiers at different echelons degraded the effectiveness of units and compromised the ability of soldiers to resist the stresses of combat (Hauser, 1973; Gabriel and Savage, 1978). Beginning in 1979, initiatives in recruiting, leadership, manning policy, and support for families reflected the interest of commanders in fostering cohesion and mutual trust and respect across ranks (Kirkland, 1987; Marlowe, et al. 1987). These reforms made fundamental changes in the ways in which military personnel behave toward each other.

One of the reforms in the field of leadership, the after action review (AAR), illustrates the readiness of military leaders to embrace psychologically constructive innovations. AARs were conceived as a means of improving performance by convening all of the participants in a combat or training event immediately after the event to go over it minute by minute to see what worked, what failed, and why. Following a model established by the Wehrmacht (the German Army in World War II) after the invasion of Poland in 1939, everyone was to be on an equal footing, and recriminations were not permitted (Murray, 1980). Although AARs are intended primarily to get members of units into an active learning posture, they also strengthen trust and cohesion within units. AARs have the potential to be a form of critical incident debriefing effective both as a palliative for acute stress symptoms and as a prophylactic against chronic disorders. The chapters by Belenky and Martin, Humphrey, and Pecano and Hickey demonstrate the efficacy of such debriefings. During Operation Just Cause, the U.S. invasion of Panama in 1989, no divisional mental health teams deployed. However, soldiers reported that when AARs were conducted, they helped alleviate stress (Kirkland et al., 1996).

By August 1990, when Saddam Hussein's forces invaded Kuwait, many of the reforms in the human dimensions had taken firm root in the military culture. Recruiters had brought in smart soldiers, manning policies kept them together, and realistic, challenging training built trust and cohesion (Kittfield, 1995). Leaders learned that telling their troops the truth, and progressively empowering them, would lead to their committing their intellectual and emotional as well as their physical resources to accomplishing the mission. While command was changing the nature of human interactions in line units, the Army Medical Department and the Army Staff were studying the problems of preventing, and providing forward treatment for, combat stress symptoms. Stokes's chapter describes how line and medical staff officers, working in the context of forecasts of future war, developed doctrine and organization for forward treatment during fast moving operations.

Prevention of combat stress disorder was a high priority because in a small professional army, a soldier can expect to see combat more than once in a single enlistment and several times in a career.   Whereas in a conscript army, veterans—with their combat stress disorders—were discharged at the ends of their terms of service, in a professional army they stay in. Management of posttraumatic stress disorders becomes the responsibility of the Army rather than the civil sector. Moreover, military psychiatrists learned from studies of the Yom Kippur War in Israel in 1973 that even a brief exposure to combat can produce acute and/or chronic stress disorders and that the effects of exposure to the stresses of combat are cumulative.   Contrary to conventional wisdom that repeated exposure to combat makes soldiers battle hardened, some veterans have proved to be more vulnerable to combat stress breakdown than those exposed for the first time (Adler, 1994).   In a professional army, effective management of the stresses imposed by combat is a component of the psychological readiness of the force.

Of the many issues considered during the Army Medical System Program Review in 1984–1985, one of the most important was establishing the credibility of medical combat stress control in the minds of line soldiers. Research conducted following Operation Just Cause made it clear that commanders and soldiers alike mistrusted mental health staffs. By contrast, chaplains enjoyed strong acceptance (Kirkland and Ender, 1991). The program review specified that the Army Medical Department was to build credibility by assigning experienced rather than junior personnel to mental health positions in divisions, training those personnel in basic soldier skills so they could operate in the field with their supported units, and directing division mental health staffs to give priority in peacetime to training with their supported units rather than augmenting garrison mental health sections. Psychiatrists, psychologists, social workers, and behavioral science specialists were to be active consultants to commanders and were to be visible and useful in peacetime so they could be trusted in wartime.

The experiences recounted in this book tell how some mental health professionals overcame obstacles to achieve these goals, and how others were overcome by them. Leading Part I, Stokes provides the background for mental health operations throughout the Army. Cline describes efforts to maintain mental health services for troops left behind in Germany, and for the families of those who deployed, while organizing a battle fatigue reconditioning unit for soldiers evacuated from the theater of operations. Martin and Fagan relate the history of the build up of Army combat stress control capabilities in Saudi Arabia, and Ragan describes the development of mental health resources for the Marines. Holsenbeck and Ruck were members of the 528th Medical Detachment, the only unit in the Active Army dedicated to combat stress control. Their two chapters provide a perspective on mental health operations in the fast moving XVIII Airborne Corps.

Campbell and Engel's chapter tells the story of organizing a divisional mental health team in the continental U.S. (CONUS) based 1st Cavalry Division; Sutton and Clark tell about the process in the 1st Armored Division based in Germany.

Conducting combat stress control during the war is the focus of the chapters in Part II. Belenky, Martin, and Marcy, two of whom improvised a combat stress control team to support the 2nd Armored Cavalry Regiment, offer a set of combat stress case studies. Humphrey, a psychiatric nurse who organized a team of chaplains to conduct debriefings with the victims of a SCUD missile attack, tells about the problems of improvising combat stress control on an ad hòc basis. Pecano and Hickey report on a support unit in the 1st Infantry Division afflicted with combat stress symptoms as a consequence of accidental deaths just after the fighting ended. Dinneen, who served on a Navy hospital ship, demonstrates the ripple effects of trauma following a boiler explosion on the *Iwo Jima*. The survivors of the explosion, the other crew members on the stricken ship, and the medical personnel who worked in vain to save many of the victims all needed post trauma debriefings. Laedtke, an occupational therapist assigned to a Corps level mental health unit, provides a detailed description of the use of occupational therapy in the treatment of combat stress reaction.

Part III is devoted to research and review of lessons learned. Gifford and his colleagues from the Department of Military Psychiatry of the Walter Reed Army Institute of Research report on their studies of cohesion conducted in the field during the build up and the war. Martin and Cline summarize the findings of a postwar conference on the lessons learned from the Persian Gulf War with respect to combat psychiatry. Belenky and Martin review what worked and show where additional thinking and effort are required.

OPERATION DESERT SHIELD

The title of the official history of the Persian Gulf War, *Certain Victory* (Scales, 1994), belies the physical strain and psychological stress the soldiers endured while holding the line against Saddam Hussein and ultimately driving his army out of Kuwait. From the psychological perspective, soldiers facing the Iraqi Army during the six months from August 1990 through February 1991 knew they were outnumbered, outgunned, and faced chemical weapons against which they were not sure they had an adequate defense. They were exposed in a desert. Temperatures ranged from murderously hot to freezing in the course of a day; fine sand penetrated every crevice of their weapons, equipment, and bodies; scorpions and other fauna were capable of inflicting near mortal stings; and they could rarely bathe (Scales, 1994, pp.119–21). They were defending a country (Saudi Arabia) with a strange and hostile culture. Ordinary aspects of American culture, such as drinking alcohol, women's clothing and deportment, and numerous religious faiths, were mortally sinful in the eyes of the Saudis. But the most severe source of stress was the probability that the Iraqis would attack the thin U.S. forces in overwhelming strength.

The Iraqis invaded Kuwait on August 2nd and organized defensive positions along the frontier with Saudi Arabia. By August 14th the 2nd Brigade of the 82nd Airborne Division, with 4575 soldiers and zero tanks, faced eight Iraqi divisions with 140,000 soldiers and 1100 tanks. During the next two months, the 1st Marine Division, the 101st Air Assault Division, the 24th Mechanized Infantry Division, the rest of the 82nd Airborne Division, the 12th Aviation Brigade, the British 7th Armored Brigade, and the Saudi Eastern Area Command arrived and took up positions. Together they had 1123 tanks. Concurrently, the Iraqis deployed 22 divisions with 3790 tanks into the Kuwaiti theater of operations (Scales, 1994, pp. 96–97, 144). Those were tense weeks. Not until October 22, with the arrival of the 1st Cavalry Division, did the Coalition Forces have a realistic capability to defend themselves and Saudi Arabia against an Iraqi attack.

The Iraqis had a large, modern artillery arm capable of firing chemical and biological weapons as well as high explosives. Iraqi officers and non-commissioned officers (NCOs) had eight years of recent combat experience, whereas only a handful of American leaders had participated in the week long invasion of Grenada or the 48 hour invasion of Panama. The Iraqis had six months and 540,000 men to organize defensive positions, harden communications, install obstacles, plant mines, prepare fire trenches, and rehearse defensive maneuvers without interruption by the Coalition Forces. The Iraqi command, control and air defense communication systems were modern, well protected, and redundant (Gordon and Trainor, 1995).

Even in February 1991, when the U.S. VII Corps had arrived and 35 nations had sent contingents, the coalition still had but 17 divisions (nine U.S., three Egyptian, one Syrian, one United Kingdom, one French, and two division equivalents from the Gulf states), with 3360 tanks facing 42 Iraqi divisions with 4280 tanks (Blair, 1992, pp. 120,128). It is worth remembering that the German Wehrmacht had only 2574 tanks when it defeated the French, British, Dutch, and Belgian Armies in May–June 1940 (Guderian, 1952, p. 472).

The sources of stress were abundant, but the resources for managing it were limited. Central Command (CENTCOM), the U.S. joint headquarters responsible for all operations in the Middle Eastern theater, assigned priority for transportation to combat forces, so support units such as medical detachments were slow to arrive. Second, independent brigades and rear area service units had no mental health staff authorized. Finally, the majority of positions in division mental health sections and mental health detachments in CONUS were not filled in peacetime. These units and sections had to organize themselves using reservists, the Professional Officer Filler System (PROFIS), levies on hospitals, and personnel assigned direct from schools (See Table 1).

Table 1
Professional Staffing of Divisional Mental Health Sections

Division	Psychiatrist	Psychologist	Social Worker
82nd Airborne	PROFIS	Exp., good cred.	New
101 Air Aslt.	PROFIS	PROFIS (applied to retire)	New
24th Mech. Inf.	PROFIS	Exp., but no field exp.	New
1st Cavalry	PROFIS	PROFIS	Exp., good cred.
1st Mech. Inf.	Levied	Some experience	Levied
1st Armored	Exp. (Sinai)	Levied	New
3rd Armored	Exp. (hosp. only)	Experienced	Experienced

Note: Exp = experienced.; cred. = credibility with line soldiers.

Sutton and Clark make it clear that members of the hurriedly organized mental health teams were themselves at high risk for stress disorders because they did not know each other, knew little of their roles, and were strangers in the units they supported.

OPERATION DESERT STORM, THE PLAN

The U.S. Central Command (CENTCOM) began planning for an aerial attack on Iraqi forces in mid-August, and laid the foundations for a ground offensive a month later. On October 31st President George Bush approved deploying forces capable of defeating the Iraqi Army, liberating Kuwait, and destroying eight divisions of the Republican Guard, the military foundation of Saddam Hussein's power. It took six months to assemble the ground forces, but aviation assets were available several weeks earlier.

The air war would use Army, Navy, Air Force, and Marine Corps aviation assets, but under joint operations doctrine it was planned and directed by officers of the Air Force. They had a private agenda of demonstrating that airpower could win the war alone. Aviators had sought to demonstrate that strategic bombing could win wars in 1940 (the Germans), 1944–1945 (the British and Americans), 1950–1953 (the Americans), and off and on during the war in Vietnam (the Americans), and they had failed. With laser guided bombs, they hoped finally to make their point in Iraq in 1991. They failed again, and in the process they caused severe strains in the joint service fabric of CENTCOM.

Army commanders complained about their lack of control over the selection of targets, Navy intelligence officers believed that the Iraqis had figured out that the Air Force centralized target designation system required a three day lead time and moved key equipment inside that cycle, and the Marines finally withdrew their aircraft from the joint air war. The Air Force planners pledged to destroy 50 percent of the Iraqi ground combat units, and there were endless arguments between soldiers, airmen, and Marines about how close they came. But interservice squabbling notwithstanding, the damage and casualties inflicted by the aerial assault isolated units, weakened morale, and convinced a substantial proportion of Iraqi soldiers that the war was hopeless. Many deserted or surrendered at the first opportunity. On January 29th–30th the Iraqi high command attempted to initiate a bloody ground war by invading Saudi Arabia along an 80 mile front with three armored and mechanized divisions. In the resulting battle of Khafji, two U. S. Marine light armored infantry battalions and a brigade of Saudi led Arab troops from several countries, supported by concentrated air attacks, sufficed to defeat the Iraqi corps and destroy 41 of their tanks. The battle demonstrated that any Iraqi mechanized force that sought to maneuver on either side of the Kuwaiti–Saudi Arabian border would be destroyed from the air. As a consequence, the Iraqi Army could not risk a mobile defense and had to dig its armored vehicles into the sand.

The CENTCOM ground battle plan as ultimately implemented was based on five corps sized elements. Closest to the Persian Gulf was Joint Forces Command East (JFCE), a 37,000 man pan Arab force comprising brigades and battalions from Bahrain, Bangladesh, Kuwait, Morocco, Oman, Qatar, Saudi Arabia, Senegal, and the United Arab Emirates. Commanded by Saudi Major General Sultan Ibn Al Mutairi and deployed on a 12 mile front, the mission of JFCE was to attack north along the coast.

Immediately west of JFCE was the I Marine Expeditionary Force (IMEF) under Marine Lieutenant General Walter Boomer. It comprised the 1st and 2nd Marine Divisions, the 1st Brigade of the Army 2nd Armored Division, and a Marine Air Wing. Deployed on a 55 mile front, the mission of IMEF was to attack through the two defensive belts of the Saddam Line to seize the Kuwait airport and cut off the escape of Iraqi forces in Kuwait City. As Ragan points out in his chapter, the Marines were even less well prepared to manage combat stress casualties than was the Army.

To the west of the Marines was Joint Forces Command North (JFCN), commanded by an Egyptian general. It included two Egyptian mechanized divisions and an armored division, and a Syrian armored division along the 55 miles of the Kuwaiti border. JFCN was to attack north and ultimately to liberate Kuwait City. JFCE, the Marine Expeditionary Force, and JFCN together had the strength of eight divisions. They faced 18 Iraqi divisions manning the heavily fortified Saddam Line. CENTCOM expected these three corps to be engaged in a prolonged, intense struggle while the other two corps made sweeping movements around the western flank of the Iraqi defenses to trap the Republican Guard. In the event, the effects of the aerial attack and Marine infiltration of the Iraqi defensive positions led to their rapid collapse.

At the end of G Day (the first day of the ground war, February 24), the Marines had penetrated all of the defenses and seized El Jaber airfield. At dawn on G+1, the Iraqi III Corps, which had concealed its maneuvers by hiding in the smoke from burning oil fields, counterattacked the 1st Marine Division. The

Iraqis were largely protected from air attack by the smoke, but after five hours of furious fighting the Marines prevailed. The Iraqi high command ordered a general withdrawal from Kuwait. By the morning of February 27, the Marines had secured the area around Kuwait City and the Egyptian–Syrian JFCN was on the way to liberate the city itself.

The main effort against the Republican Guard was to be made by VII Corps and XVIII Airborne Corps executing a wide sweep to the west. VII Corps occupied assembly areas to the west of JFCN on a front of 70 miles. Commanded by Lieutenant General Frederick Franks, it included the 1st Armored Division, 3rd Armored Division, 1st Mechanized Infantry Division, and 2nd Armored Cavalry Regiment of the U.S. Army and the 1st Armored Division of the British Army. Its mission was to break through the western extension of the Saddam Line, held by six Iraqi divisions, and then drive northeast 220 miles into Iraq and destroy the Republican Guard.

On the left of VII Corps was XVIII Airborne Corps under the command of Lieutenant General Gary E. Luck. Luck's corps, deployed on a 100-mile front, comprised the 24th Mechanized Infantry Division, 101st Air Assault Division, 82nd Airborne Division, and 3rd Armored Cavalry Regiment of the U.S. Army and the French 6th Light Armored Division. The mission of the corps was to advance 155 miles northeast into Iraq to the Euphrates River to isolate the Republican Guard from reinforcements and to block its escape.

The Army 1st Cavalry Division had independent missions within the eastern portion of the VII Corps zone from February 7 through February 26 (G+2). Between February 7 and February 20, it attacked Iraqi forces guarding the southern end of the Wadi al Batin, a wide stream bed that extends from well into Saudi Arabia, along the western frontier between Kuwait and Iraq, and into Iraq. The wadi is a natural avenue of approach and was the route along which the Iraqi high command expected the Coalition Forces to attack. To confirm their expectations, the Division on February 7 began a series of artillery raids, helicopter incursions, and finally a mechanized thrust by 2nd Brigade 10 miles into the wadi. The 1st Squadron of the 5th Cavalry fought a dug in and reinforced Iraqi infantry battalion and lost four armored vehicles, with four soldiers killed and nine wounded. The mission was successful in that the Iraqis kept six of their eight armored divisions positioned along the wadi. Following this deception mission, the division became the CENTCOM theater reserve until February 26, when it was attached to VII Corps for the final attack on the Republican Guard.

VII CORPS AND XVIII CORPS IN THE BATTLE

The mission of XVIII Airborne Corps required maneuvers that were, in distance and speed, unprecedented in the history of warfare. On G Day, the 101st Air Assault Division used helicopters to establish Forward Operating Base Cobra 90 miles into Iraqi territory. The air assault into the area chosen for the forward operating base entailed mounting a combined air infantry artillery attack on a dug in Iraqi battalion. The base was capable of providing logistical support for attack helicopters operating over a 150 mile radius, of supporting ground combat operations by helicopter borne forces in the Euphrates valley 60 miles further into Iraq, and of launching the next forward operating base. Concurrent with the air assault, the division dispatched a 1400-truck, 90 mile-long ground convoy to provide the enormous amounts of fuel required for the helicopters. There was no road, but the divisional engineers improved the *Dub al Haj* (route of the pilgrim), an ancient trail just in front of the fuel trucks. Heliborne scouts had located and eliminated Iraqi Army outposts along the trail during the preceding week.

The weather on February 24 and 25 included dense fog, heavy rain, and wind blown dust that made flying almost impossible and that turned the dry, dusty desert into a sea of deep, sticky mud. But by the night of G+1, the division had established roadblocks in battalion strength on Highway 8 paralleling the Euphrates River. The next day, the force was built up to brigade strength, defeated all Iraqi units in the area, and sealed off Iraqi forces in the Kuwaiti theater of operations from reinforcement from or escape to the west. On G+3, the division established Forward Operating Base Viper 50 miles east of Cobra to support helicopter attacks on Iraqi forces around Basrah. On G+4, the 101st suffered its only casualties when a medical evacuation helicopter was shot down. Five crew members died and three, including a female flight surgeon, were seriously injured and captured.

While the 101st Division was seizing bases in Iraq by aerial assault, 3rd Armored Cavalry Regiment (ACR) and the 24th Mechanized Infantry Division replicated the 101st's moves on a somewhat shorter radius on the ground. Rolling day and night with three brigades abreast on a 40 mile front, the division reached the Euphrates River Valley on G+2 and charged east down Highway 8. That night, a troop of the 3rd ACR accidentally got into a firefight with an engineer battalion from VII Corps. One soldier was killed and another wounded. The 3rd ACR had no organic mental health element, and Ruck in his chapter describes how the 528th Medical Detachment sought to train its medics and leaders in combat stress control techniques.

On G+3, the 24th Division assaulted Jalibah airfield, destroying an Iraqi tank battalion. During the battle, two U.S. battalions got intermingled and fired on each other. Two soldiers were killed and eight wounded. Later in the day, one brigade of the division seized Tallil Airfield, one of the most heavily defended installations in Iraq. The bulk of the division, including the 3rd ACR, raced eastward fighting elements of the Nebuchadnezzar, Al Faw, and Adnan Republican Guard Divisions. By G+4, the 24th Division was within 30 miles of Basrah.

The deep incursions into enemy territory by the 101st and 24th Divisions were possible because their left flank was covered by the French 6th Light Armored Division reinforced by elements of the U.S. 82nd Airborne Division. This team defeated the 45th Infantry Division, the principal Iraqi force west of the Saddam

Line, and blocked Iraqi action against the vulnerable resupply line along the *Dub al Haj*.

VII Corps was the most powerful force in CENTCOM, with four (after G+3, five) heavy divisions. In conjunction with the Air Force, it was to destroy the Republican Guard. To deceive the Iraqis about the direction of the main attack, VII Corps was to cross the Iraqi border one day after I Marine Expeditionary Force and XVIII Corps launched their attacks. But the Marines' success upset the CENTCOM plan because it accelerated the withdrawal of Iraqi units and made it possible that the Republican Guard might escape north of the Euphrates before the flanking attack by VII Corps could catch it. Realizing in the first hours of the attack that the Marines would advance much more rapidly than expected, CENTCOM ordered VII Corps to attack 12 hours earlier than originally planned. It met the challenge.

The 2nd Armored Cavalry Regiment was to lead the Corps for the first two days. The 2nd ACR crossed the Iraqi border west of the Saddam Line, and when the order to go early came down, it was already six miles into Iraq. Advancing on a 25 mile front with helicopter scouts in front followed by a line of Bradley armored infantry vehicles and then a line of Abrams tanks, it penetrated 30 miles by nightfall while defeating a brigade of the Iraqi 26th Division. In the late afternoon of G-Day, the U.S. 1st and 3rd Armored Divisions followed the 2nd ACR north. Concurrently, the 1st Mechanized Infantry Division assaulted the western end of the Saddam Line held by the Iraqi 48th Division and the bulk of the 26th Division. Using a massive artillery barrage followed by armored combat earthmovers and tanks fitted with mine plows, in two hours the division made a breach that had been expected to require 18 hours.

On G+1, the British 1st Armored Division surged through the gap cut by the 1st Infantry Division and destroyed the Iraqi 52nd Armored Division. The 1st U.S. Armored Division captured the last brigade of the Iraqi 26th Division and surrounded the town of al Busayyah. At noon the 2nd ACR, leading the advance, met a brigade of the Iraqi 12th Armored Division. Although the 2nd ACR was not supposed to engage in heavy combat, its gunners destroyed the brigade in 20 minutes.

In the midafternoon of G+2, the 2nd ACR met the 18th Brigade, Tawakalna Mechanized Division of the Republican Guard in the Battle of 73 Easting. In six minutes, the 2nd Squadron of the 2nd ACR destroyed 37 T-72 tanks and 15 armored infantry vehicles. That night, two Bradley armored infantry vehicles of the 2nd ACR fired on each other, wounding six Americans. Martin and Fagin, researchers from the Walter Reed Army Institute of Research, tell in their chapter how they and a reserve psychiatrist cobbled together a combat stress control team to support the 2nd ACR. Also during the night, the 1st Armored Division fought the 29th Brigade of the Tawakalna Division destroying 76 T-72 tanks and 103 other armored vehicles while losing only four of its own Abrams tanks. One

Abrams was hit twice, but its internal compartmentation and fire suppression systems enabled all of the crew members to survive.

In the afternoon of G+2 the 3rd Armored Division began a close-in fight with dug-in infantry and armor of the 9th Brigade of the Tawakalna. The battle went on all night as the Iraqis put up a tenacious defense. The division inflicted heavy losses on the Iraqis, but three friendly fire incidents destroyed four Bradleys and killed four soldiers. The 1st Mechanized Infantry Division, which had begun fighting four days before G Day and never stopped, relieved the 2nd ACR and fought a brigade of the Iraqi 12th Armored Division until daybreak. The 1st Brigade destroyed more than 100 armored vehicles for the loss of two Bradleys, but the 3rd Brigade lost five Abrams tanks, five Bradleys, and six soldiers to friendly fire. Management of the stress engendered by one of these incidents is described by Pecano and Hickey.

At dawn on G+3, the 1st Armored Division advanced on the Medina Armored Division of the Republican Guard with 350 Abrams tanks. In the five hour Battle of Medina Ridge, the largest tank battle of the Gulf War, the 1st Armored destroyed 300 tanks and armored infantry vehicles for a loss of two Bradleys and one soldier. One Abrams engaged four T-72 tanks and destroyed them all before any of them could get off a shot. A Bradley crew, using three different weapon systems, killed an armored infantry vehicle, a group of running soldiers, another armored infantry vehicle, a T-72 tank, and a third armored infantry vehicle in less than a minute.

All of the divisions of XVIII and VII Corps were poised to attack on the morning of G+4, and 1st Armored Division destroyed another 100 of the Medina Division's armored vehicles before the cease fire went into effect at 0800. The Iraqi forces remaining in Kuwait withdrew, and the 1st and 3rd U.S. Armored Divisions, the 1st Mechanized Infantry Division, and the British 1st Armored Division drove on to the Persian Gulf.

In southern Iraq, units of the XVIII Airborne Corps held their positions as Iraqi units streamed north from Kuwait. Sporadic fire fell on U.S. units, but they maintained fire discipline. The tempo of the fire increased on G+6 (March 2nd), and about 200 Iraqi armored vehicles of the Hammurabi Armored Division of the Republican Guard charged across the front of 1st Brigade of the 24th Mechanized Infantry Division while firing at its forward elements. The brigade commander used artillery and helicopter gunships to knock out the vehicles at the front and rear of the Iraqi column and then destroyed every vehicle—185 tanks and armored infantry vehicles, 400 trucks, and 34 artillery pieces. There were no friendly casualties in this action, but U.S. soldiers continued to suffer casualties from unexploded bomblets that littered Iraq and Kuwait.

CONCLUSION

Operation Desert Storm demonstrated marked differences between policies and practice for managing physical casualties and those for managing stress casualties. The first difference is in the relative emphasis accorded to prevention as compared to treatment. While preventive medicine is vital to support the health of the force, it can do little to limit casualties caused by shot and shell. With stress casualties, prevention begins the day the soldier joins up and is continued by commanders, chaplains, and mental health professionals up to and into the battle. Mental health professionals need to be up front training soldiers and leaders in managing their own and their comrades' stress reactions and conducting critical incident debriefings.

The second difference is in the locus of treatment and the direction of movement. Physical casualties are evacuated as quickly as possible to a definitive care facility in the rear areas of the theater or outside the theater. There is no expectation that they will return to duty during the conflict in which they were wounded, were injured, or became ill. Combat stress casualties, on the other hand, are to be treated as far forward as possible and returned to their units within 24 to 72 hours. Stress casualties in divisional units are to be treated no farther back than the brigade support area.

These divergent policies presage a continued diminution of the number of medical personnel and the range of medical expertise required in the division and corps areas. It is important that mental health staff not be caught up in this trend. For combat stress control to be effective, the numbers and the skills have to be close to the supported units. Rapid return to duty conserves the fighting strength of the units and also provides the best prognosis for the individual. Experience in the Persian Gulf War indicates a need for augmentation of the mental health staff at division and the development of a combat stress control capability in the brigade.

As you read this book, you will discern three themes. The first is that when commanders accept the fact that the stresses of making war affect soldiers in all types of units in all wars, their efforts to build competence, trust, and cohesion will minimize the incidence of combat stress casualties. The second theme is that when the Army Medical Department organizes, staffs, equips, and trains deployable, qualified stress control teams to teach stress management techniques and to debrief soldiers who have experienced traumatic events, stress casualties can be prevented or restored quickly to duty. The third theme is that commanders' action to sustain morale, chaplains' action to provide spiritual aid, and mental health professionals' action to control combat stress reactions are complementary. They make their greatest contributions to the well being of the soldier and to the psychological readiness of the force when they work in concert.

REFERENCES

Adler, A. (1994). *Post-Traumatic Stress Symptoms in U.S. Veterans in the Gulf War.* U.S. Army Medical Research Unit-Europe Report #20: Heidelburg, Germany.

Blair, A. (1992). *At War in the Gulf War: A Chronology.* College Station, Texas: Texas A&M University Press.

Dunnigan, J. and R. Macedonia. (1993). *Getting It Right: American Military Reforms to the Gulf War and Beyond.* New York: William Morrow.

Gabriel, R. and P. Savage. (1978). *Crisis in Command: Mismanagement in the Army.* New York: Hill and Wang.

Gordon, M. and B. Trainor. (1995). *The Generals' War: The Inside Story of the Conflict in the Gulf.* Boston: Little, Brown and Co.

Guderian, H. (1952). *Panzer Leader.* Trans. by C. Fitzgibbon. New York: E. P. Dutton.

Hauser, W. (1973). *America's Army in crisis: A Study in Civil-Military Relations.* Baltimore: John's Hopkins University Press.

Kirkland, F. (1987). *Leading in COHORT Companies.* WRAIR Report NP 88 13 (ADA 192886). Washington, D.C.: Walter Reed Army Institute of Research.

Kirkland, F. (1990). "The gap between leadership policy and practice: A historical perspective." *Parameters,* XX (3):50–62.

Kirkland, F. and M. Ender. (1991). *Analysis of Interview Data from Operation Just Cause.* Working paper. Washington, D.C.: Department of Military Psychiatry, Walter Reed Army Institute of Research.

Kirkland, F., M. Ender, R. Gifford, K. Wright and D. Marlowe. (1996). "Human dimensions of rapid force projection." *Mil. Rev.,* LXXVI (2), in press.

Kittfield, J. (1995). *Prodigal Soldiers.* New York: Simon & Schuster.

Marlowe, D., F. Kirkland, T. Furukawa, J. Teitelbaum, L. Ingraham, and B. Caine. (1987). *Unit Manning System Field Evaluation: Technical Report No. 5* (ADA 207193). Washington, D.C.: Walter Reed Army Institute of Research.

Meyer, E. and R. Ancel. (1995). *Who Will Lead?* Westport, Conn.: Praeger.

Murray, W. (1981). "The German response to victory in Poland." *Armed Forces and Society,* VII (2): 285–298.

Scales, R. (1994). *Certain Victory: The U.S. Army in the Gulf War.* Washington: Brassey's.

Acknowledgments

This book represents a difficult journey that began with our deployment to the Gulf War and eventually took us through a series of life events that have included personal loss, serious illness, retirement, and career change. We are thankful for the encouragement we have received from our families and friends. Without their support, we would never have completed this task. We dedicate this book to the men and women who served in the Gulf War and their families.

We wish to gratefully acknowledge the continuous support of Colonel C.F. Tyner and David H. Marlowe. Colonel Tyner's leadership while Director of the Walter Reed Army Institute of Research, and Dr. Marlowe's guidance while Chief of the Institute's Department of Military Psychiatry, have encouraged and sustained this work. They have been wonderful mentors and thoughtful colleagues.

Part I

MENTAL HEALTH SERVICES IN THE THEATER OF OPERATIONS

U.S. Army Mental Health System: Divisional and Corps Level Mental Health Units

James W. Stokes

INTRODUCTION

This chapter describes the historical development of the mental health sections in Army combat divisions and the specialized mental health detachments assigned as corps- and theater-level mental health resources. It also compares the mental health assets actually sent to Southwest Asia for the Gulf War with what the organizational plan embodied in obsolescent Tables of Organization and Equipment (TO&E) and with new, updated doctrine and new TO&Es. The new doctrine and organization had been under development since 1983 to correct identified deficiencies and to update units to the conditions of the modern, mobile, fluid, and deep battlefield. This chapter has two parts: a discussion of division level mental health and a discussion of corps level mental health. Each part provides background information concerning the structure of mental health assets in general and as they were in the Gulf War theater of operations.

DIVISION LEVEL MENTAL HEALTH STRUCTURE

Background

During World War I, a trained psychiatrist was assigned to each combat division. Following World War II and during the Korean War, the psychiatrist was augmented with a social work officer, a clinical psychologist, and enlisted specialists (now called behavioral science specialists). In 1957, the principles of combat neuropsychiatry and the role of the organic division mental health section and its members were codified in Army Regulations (AR 40-216, Neuropsychiatry and Mental Health).

Since the Vietnam era, all U.S. Army divisions nominally have three officers (psychiatrist, psychologist, social worker) and six to eight enlisted technicians. In some divisions, such as the airborne, the mental health section was in the headquarters and support company of the medical battalion. In heavy divisions, the mental health section was a part of the main support medical company of the main support battalion. Prior to the start of the Gulf War, there were plans to convert all divisions to the main support battalion format.

Structural and Operational Deficiencies

To understand the structure of mental health services at the time of the Gulf War, it is necessary to back up a decade. In the early 1980s, the division mental health section had been successfully defended during a series of arbitrary personnel cuts in the number of medical slots allowed in divisions. However, several deficiencies were noted in division mental health capability during the Army's 1982 Medical Mission Area Analysis (MMAA, 1982) and a subsequent Army Medical System Program Review (MSPR, 1984–1985) initiated by General Maxwell R. Thurman, Vice Chief of Staff of the Army. The MMAA and the MSPR were major staff projects designed to modernize the Army Medical Department. They reviewed the entire Army Medical Department field deployable system—doctrine, training, organization, and equipment. They compared the current system's capabilities against the validated future threat (the Soviet threat in Europe), and they requested Department of Army approval to correct noted deficiencies. General Thurman took a personal interest in Combat Stress Control (CSC, a.k.a. "combat psychiatry" or "combat mental health"), and during the MSPR, it was finally recognized as an autonomous Army Medical Department functional area (as are Preventive Medicine, Dentistry, and Veterinary Medicine).

One CSC deficiency was the lack of organizational ability by the division mental health section to provide a noncommissioned officer (that is, senior enlisted behavioral science specialist) and professional level preventive and triage support at the level of the combat maneuver brigades. The typical division mental health section lacked the mobility (organic tactical vehicles) and communications equipment (radios) required to send preventive and triage teams to the brigade support areas.

A second CSC deficiency was that the various TO&Es did not authorize sufficiently high rank for the division mental health behavioral science specialists. In an organized hierarchy such as the Army, sufficient rank is essential to achieve the necessary experience, credibility, and authority to function as an effective consultant to middle and senior level line and medical officers. Most of the enlisted behavioral science specialists assigned to the Gulf War division–level mental health positions lacked the rank which the TO&Es

allowed. Recommendations to correct these deficiencies were still being staffed in the Pentagon at the start of the Gulf War.

The 1984 MSPR also identified deficiencies in the training and rank of the mental health officers being assigned to division mental health positions. Lack of field skills and insufficient knowledge of the field units they supported was common. This was partly because the mental health officers had become fully committed to and preoccupied with garrison type mental health duties. Army Regulation AR 40-216 had authorized use of division mental health assets to support the community mental health service when in garrison. In practice, this translated to division mental health officers being full time "borrowed manpower" in the military hospital or community mental health clinic.

As a result, the division mental health officers had little time to provide on site command consultation in the division's work and training areas. They were even less able to participate in field exercises or staff planning efforts. Because they were not involved in the daily routine of the division medical unit, they tended to be perceived (and to perceive themselves) as outsiders and to have no claim on their vehicles or equipment. To the extent that they were never seen in the field, the rest of the division came to regard these mental health personnel as useful only in garrison. To quote General Maxwell Thurman, "the shrinks from division—they're the guys in the rear who rubber stamp the problem soldiers you want to get rid of."

Furthermore, many division psychiatrists, psychologists, and social workers were in their first utilization tour after completion of professional training and/or just finishing the Army Medical Department's Officer Basic Course. Their junior company grade rank received little respect from division or even brigade staff. They had received little formal didactic instruction in military and combat psychiatry during their training, ostensibly because other clinical topics took precedence for the program to maintain civilian accreditation. Their community or division psychiatry rotation might have given them several weeks of cumulative experience in a post or even division mental health clinic, but there they selectively saw the soldiers who were either self referred or command referred because they were not fitting in well with their units and the unit's leadership. New mental health officers had typically little knowledge of the field Army's organization, ethic, culture, or vocabulary, except from this negative perspective.

The young, junior officers put into division mental health sections struggled through their assignments performing the clinical skills they had learned in training, but they never formed the cohesive bonds or developed the military and consultation liaison skills required to make the division mental health section a functioning part of the division. When social workers or psychologists of higher experience and rank were assigned to the division, they were frequently frustrated by the Army regulation which made a junior, inexperienced psychiatrist the head of the division mental health section and spokesperson to the division surgeon and staff. Most were glad to leave the division assignment.

For years, it had been the policy at the Surgeon General's Office to give priority to filling division slots before garrison Medical Activity positions. However, in the late 1980s, there was an Army wide shortage of psychiatrists and clinical psychologists relative to the positions which needed filling. Mental health care costs made up a substantial percentage of ever rising health care costs. The Surgeon General's consultants made the decision, in some cases, to give priority to assignment in the installation hospital clinical service rather than to the division mental health section at the same post. The hospital medical commander would then have to identify someone (usually the same newly assigned mental health officer) to be the PROFIS (Professional Officer Filler System) assignee to go to that division if (but only if) the division was deployed to combat. This had the virtue of at least calling things the way they were—the division mental health officers were being full time borrowed manpower in the peacetime garrison medical care system anyway. However, it had the adverse effect of severing even the tenuous, nominal ties that mental health officers gained from the division staff and from the rest of the division mental health section by wearing the distinctive division patch on their left shoulder sleeve.

Combat Stress Control within the Division

In the late 1980s, field manuals were being written and staffed which provided doctrine for how the division mental health sections should function. First was draft FM 8-15-1, Health Service Support in the Airborne, Air Assault, and Light Division (published as a draft in August 1986 and still operative in draft form in 1991). The detailed paragraph 5-25 for the division mental health sections specified that one senior noncommissioned officer (NCO) behavioral science specialist (exact rank not specified) should be allocated by the consolidated division mental health section to support each maneuver brigade as its Brigade CSC Coordinator. That NCO's duties were carefully spelled out in the manual. The mental health officers were expected to work together routinely at the main support medical company and thus to make unique, professional skills available to the whole division. They were to come forward frequently to mentor, supervise, and provide professional-level skill at the brigades whenever appropriate.

The role of the Brigade Combat Stress Control Coordinator (behavioral science specialist NCO) and the reinforcing division mental health officers was described in the Combat Stress Control appendix in Army FM 8-10-5, Division/Brigade Surgeon's Handbook. This was circulating for staffing in the divisions as a final draft when the Gulf War occurred. The CSC appendix was printed and distributed by mail to mental health personnel in the Persian Gulf as a small booklet of official interim doctrine. It arrived just before the start of the ground combat phase of the Gulf War (January 1991).

The first coordinating draft of FM 8-51, *Combat Stress Control in a Theater of Operations*, was sent out for staffing in February 1990. This manual dealt more with the corps level CSC units that could reinforce the division mental health sections than with the sections themselves, but it provided additional detail for how the division mental health section should accomplish the six critical CSC mission functions: preventive consultation, reconstitution support, neuropsychiatric triage, stabilization, restoration (one to three day forward treatment) and reconditioning (one to two week rearward treatment).

Deployment of Division Mental Health Sections during the Gulf War

What follows is an overview of unit status across division mental health sections in the predeployment and mobilization phase of the Gulf War. It is not a detailed history of every unit. Some of the units involved are discussed in greater detail in later chapters of this book. This chapter records what and who were deployed to Southwest Asia. The chapter does not assign blame to individuals for problems experienced in the process. These problems are systemic, and they deserve systemic solutions.

The 82nd Airborne Division, Fort Bragg, North Carolina. The 82nd Airborne was the first division alerted and deployed. Its psychologist had been with the division since before Operation Just Cause and had good credibility, although little opportunity for field experience. The division social work officer had just arrived at the 82nd after completing the Army Medical Department Officer Advanced Course (OAC). At OAC, he had been well briefed in the evolving CSC concept and in the experience from Operation Just Cause. The division psychiatrist position, however, was unfilled, and a PROFIS psychiatrist from the Fort Bragg hospital was assigned to fill this position. He was young and had no prior military experience. The 82nd Airborne mental health officers hustled and got themselves and some of their authorized behavioral science specialists deployed by echelons with the lead brigades. The psychiatrist followed, but he was later allowed to rotate home to take his professional board examinations. He was replaced by a volunteer psychiatrist who, although only a recent graduate of the psychiatry residency program, had used the time to become jump qualified—a highly positive credibility factor in an airborne division. The modified table of organization and equipment (MTO&E) of the airborne division did not assure that the division mental health section would have vehicles under circumstances where vehicles were in very short supply. This was the case during the initial phase of this deployment, and it greatly hampered implementation of mental health consultation and combat stress control activities during the ground combat phase of this deployment.

The 101st Air Assault Division, Fort Campbell, Kentucky.   The 101st also deployed very hastily. Its mental health section illustrated a number of the problems of the existing system. The social worker was newly assigned; the PROFIS psychiatrist (a recent residency graduate) was dual hatted as chief of inpatient psychiatry at the understaffed installation hospital; and the PROFIS psychologist had been the division psychologist earlier but was now chief of Psychology Service in the installation hospital and had already filed for retirement. That action was suspended by an Army policy designed to prevent personnel losses for the duration of the mobilization, and he was deployed.

24th Infantry Division (Mechanized), Fort Stewart, Georgia. The 24th was hastily deployed from Fort Stewart, Georgia, but its equipment and a few of its personnel traveled slowly by sea while the bulk of the personnel flew to Saudi Arabia to off load the ships when they arrived. The psychologist had been with the unit for a while but had no field experience. The social work officer was a new Army officer. She had just completed the Army Medical Department Officer Basic Course, where she had been familiarized with the evolving CSC concept. The psychiatrist, although relatively senior in rank, was a PROFIS filler from the installation hospital with no prior division or field experience. Some of the enlisted behavioral science specialists were levies from distant installations (including, by chance, one exceptionally well trained and qualified instructor from the behavioral science specialist course at the Academy of Health Sciences, Fort Sam Houston, who had worked with this author in several field exercises of the CSC concept with reserve units).

The 1st Cavalry (Cav) Division, Fort Hood, Texas. The 1st Cav had the advantage of about a month in which to pack and ship its equipment by sea and then follow by air. It also had the advantage of a social work officer who had previously been a decorated Marine infantryman and NCO in Vietnam. Later he had become a social worker specializing in Vietnam veteran counseling and the treatment of delayed postcombat post-traumatic stress disorder. He had been with the division for about 10 months and had high credibility and skill in consultation liaison. He mentored the recent residency graduate psychiatrist, the PROFIS psychologist (who had previously been a division psychologist before moving into the installation hospital), and the units' behavioral science specialists. When the division mental health section deployed, it not only had vehicles, but also radios which were not authorized by TO&E.

The 1st Infantry Division (Mechanized), Fort Riley, Kansas. The 1st Infantry Division was deployed several months later than the divisions previously discussed. Its psychologist had developed some cohesion with the unit, but the psychiatrist, social worker and many of the enlisted behavioral science specialists were levied out of installation hospital jobs.

1st Armored Division, Germany. In Europe, the 1st Armored Division had been in the process of deactivating when it received the unexpected mission to deploy to the Persian Gulf. The division psychiatrist had good training in military and unit psychiatry during her residency and had expanded on it as the invited psychiatrist with a light infantry battalion on peace keeping duty in the Sinai for six months. However, she had few mental health assets to work with initially. The four behavioral science specialists were junior and two of them just out of school. The system would not allow senior behavioral science specialists who had previously served in the division but who were now in 7th Medical Command (serving in Army hospitals in Germany) to volunteer to deploy with the division to the Persian Gulf. A division psychologist was cross attached from another division in Europe. The social work officer was assigned with the cross attached mechanized infantry brigade of another division. He had recently arrived in Europe on a permanent change of station, his family was still in transit and housing was uncertain.

3rd Armored Division, Germany. The 3rd Armored Division psychiatrist was well trained, but the majority of his time was devoted to clinical work at the regional hospital. While the social worker and psychologist were available, the division did not have its complement of behavioral science specialists. The section had not drawn its unit equipment; nor had it participated in any major divisional field training.

Independent Brigade Sized Units. Two Armored Cavalry Regiments (ACRs)—the 3rd ACR from Fort Bliss, Texas, and the 2nd ACR from Germany—deployed to the Gulf War with no organic mental health assets, even though their wartime configuration made them the size of a peacetime division. The same was basically true for the 2nd Armored Division (Forward), a brigade sized unit deployed from Germany. It had two junior behavioral science specialists, but they had only worked in garrison clinic settings and had never functioned in a division mental health section role.

Most of the division mental health sections arrived in Saudi Arabia deficient in personnel, appropriate training, supplies, and equipment. They all had a great deal to overcome. There was sufficient time before the start of the ground war to fix many problems, but lack of readiness prevented some of the sections from adequately supporting their divisions during the prolonged Desert Shield phase of the Gulf War.

CORPS LEVEL MENTAL HEALTH (OM) TEAMS

Background

The second level of mental health support in the theater of operations is the corps-level mobile stress control unit (designated by the letters "OM" and refered to as an OM team). The first U.S. Army psychiatric units— Neurological Hospitals 1, 2 and 3—were organized in World War I. These were not mobile and were located in French barracks buildings close behind the front.

In World War II, equivalent Neuropsychiatry Centers served each field Army. These were 250 cot clearing companies augmented with mental health personnel and commanded by a psychiatrist. They were not very mobile.

Based on post–World War II recommendations, the Army created a TO&E medical psychiatry detachment during the Korean War, called the KO team. Although K series teams are, by definition, hospital augmentation detachments (for example, neurosurgery or ophthalmologic surgery teams), the KO team had a very different mission. It was 100 percent mobile, with trucks, jeeps, and enough tents for its own staff and a few patients. Its psychiatrists, psychologist, social work officers, and enlisted specialists could reinforce division mental health sections or provide area. When battle conditions produced many combat exhaustion or battle fatigue cases, the KO team could roll into a medical clearing company to give it expertise in battle fatigue restoration or reconditioning, and perhaps even take it over and make the medical clearing company into a dedicated neuropsychiatry center.

Two KO teams were deployed during the Vietnam conflict. The Vietnam conflict was unlike the artillery heavy and often mechanized linear warfare of the World War II Italian and European theaters, where the KO team was conceived, or the artilleryheavy, static trench warfare of the late Korean War where it was first tested. Instead, Vietnam was predominantly a counter insurgency and midintensity counterguerrilla war with no front lines. Unit fire bases were relatively secure, and the few battle fatigue casualties produced by grueling patrols and brief but sometimes intense battles and ambushes could be rested and returned to duty in their own units.

More dramatic psychiatric cases could be whisked by medical air ambulances, like the wounded, directly from the battlefield to the combat zone hospitals, bypassing the battalion aide stations, the divisional medical companies, and the divisional mental health section officers and enlisted specialists. Meanwhile, the ambiguity and frustration of fighting a guerrilla terrorist enemy in a distant, alien culture combined with the home front problems of racial tension, drug using counterculture, and antiwar movement produced an epidemic of misconduct stress behaviors, including serious breaches of discipline and substance abuse.

Development of the OM Team Concept

As the United States withdrew from Vietnam in the early 1970s, the KO team TO&E was modified into the Medical Detachment, Psychiatric (OM team). Documentation of the reasoning behind the changes is not available. The change in the letter designation code should have clarified the role of the unit. An O series team (unlike the K series hospital augmentation detachments) was a unit which had a medical area support mission and was expected to operate autonomously. Other examples in the O series were the OA, OB, and OC Teams, which were small, medium and large medical dispensaries, respectively.

However, the major structural change involved in converting from a KO to OM team concept was to remove the inpatient psychiatric ward from the Evacuation Hospital and General Hospital TO&Es and add it to the old KO team. The addition of psychiatric nurses and psychiatric technicians to the field mobile, area-support units had good rationale. Their expertise would enable treatment of more drug and alcohol or other organic mental disorders (such as might be encountered in nuclear, biological, and chemical [NBC] scenarios) in the nonhospital, forward deployed setting which provided the best possibility for rapid return to duty. Psychiatric nurses had also proved very effective in treating conventional stress casualties in World War I.

The rationale for taking the inpatient psychiatric capability out of every combat zone and theater hospital is less clear. Perhaps the idea was that the promise of rapid stabilization with antipsychotic or sedative drugs, plus transoceanic air evacuation, had made having psychiatric inpatient wards in many theater hospitals unnecessary. If a psychiatric ward was found to be needed, then an OM team could be attached to one hospital to make it the neuropsychiatric referral center, just as another hospital might have a neurosurgery or ophthalmologic surgery detachment added to make it the center for that specialty.

The alert reader will have noticed that this concept has just confounded the mobile area support mission of the newly renamed OM team. It has been turned into a true hospital augmentation (K series) unit. That is how the OM teams appear to have been regarded by their higher headquarters and by their own members through the late 1970s and early 1980s. In any case, no one wrote any doctrine for how to use the new OM team in its combat psychiatric or stress control role.

Finally, although in the third quarter of 1971, sixty one percent of all medical evacuations from Vietnam had been psychiatric (many drug and alcohol related), and although the inpatient psychiatric wards in theater had just been transferred to OM teams, the basis of allocation rule for deploying OM teams to a theater of operation was written into the TO&E as one per 140,000 troops without organic mental health support. Since the combat divisions did have their own organic mental health sections and were therefore excluded from the accounting, this meant that even a very large corps would be entitled to only one OM team.

In fact, only one numbered active component OM team was created. This was the 528th Medical Detachment, Psychiatric. Until its activation for deployment to Saudi Arabia in September 1991, it had never been assembled for training. Its vehicles and equipment were at Fort Benning in the care of its nominal headquarters, the 34th Medical Battalion, which maintained them and naturally used them for other missions. None of its enlisted personnel had been assigned or even designated by name. Its officers were all identified only within the Professional Officer Filler System (PROFIS).

In the PROFIS system, the medical activity (hospital) commanders at a variety of posts were obliged to specify the names of health care officers of the right specialties to fill specific positions or slots in deployable TO&E units around the country. In some cases, the officers so designated were informed by their commander, usually with the reassurance that the likelihood of their ever being mobilized was small. In other cases, the PROFIS filler was not even informed that his or her name was on the computer printout for a specific TO&E unit. In fact, when this author finally got the computer printout for the 528th Medical Detachment from the 34th Medical Battalion in 1984 and contacted the 528th's designated commander, he had not even been informed that he was allocated to the 528th. Since he had another PROFIS assignment to a major headquarters which he had been told about, he assumed the latter was where he would report on mobilization.

In the 1970s, six U.S. Army Reserve OM teams were created in Boston, Massachusetts; Baltimore, Maryland; Indianapolis, Indiana; Madison, Wisconsin; Saint Paul, Minnesota; and Los Angeles, California. Prior to 1983, none of these had been involved in significant field training. Most did their two week annual training working on the psychiatric wards and clinics of a continental U.S. (CONUS) Army clinical center or major hospital, or at the confinement facility at Fort Leavenworth—hardly the best preparation for a field combat stress prevention and treatment mission.

The Structure of OM Teams

The Medical Detachment, Psychiatric (OM team) is authorized for fifteen officers, thirty three enlisted personnel, and nine vehicles and is organized as follows: The headquarters section has a psychiatrist (lieutenant colonel) commander, a clinical psychologist (captain), a field medical assistant (first lieutenant), a psychiatric ward master as noncommissioned officer in charge, a supply sergeant, and a unit clerk. The commander has a four-wheel-drive vehicle with radio, while the rest of the headquarters has a pickup truck with trailer.

The three Mobile Consultation Sections of the OM team each have a psychiatrist, two social work officers, and six behavioral science specialists. For mobility, each consultation section has two vehicles: a one ton pickup truck with trailer and a four-wheel-drive vehicle.

The Treatment Section has a psychiatrist, two psychiatric nurses, eleven psychiatric technicians, and a behavioral science specialist. This section has a two and a half-ton truck to carry its personnel, equipment, tents and cots for a twenty patient ward.

The Medical Mission Area Analysis (1982) and Medical System Program Review (1985) identified several shortcomings in the OM teams' capabilities. First, the OM teams had insufficient mobility, carrying capacity, and flexibility for the forward deployed use which would be required by the NATO plan against the Soviet threat   The computer model which generated patient workloads projected one battle fatigue casualty for every 2.5 wounded in action in that highly intense mechanized combat. If so many soldiers could not be turned around and returned to duty in one to three days within the divisions, they would quickly overload the capabilities of many more than seven OM teams in the corps areas.

One OM team requirement was to be able to reinforce the division mental health section's behavioral science NCO or NCO officer team at each maneuver brigade support area with a four-person (two officer; two enlisted, one vehicle) team. The primary mission of this combat stress control preventive team is to prevent unnecessary evacuation of combat stress casualties by improving neuropsychiatric triage (with a psychiatrist or perhaps clinical psychologist at the medical company) and by actively assisting the combat and combat support units in resting and recovering stressed soldiers in their own combat service support trains (with a circuit riding social worker and behavioral science specialist). Similar reinforcement would be needed by any separate brigades or armored cavalry regiments which did not have their own organic mental health officers.

Next was the requirement to increase the division's capability to provide a two to three day restoration program at its main support medical company in the division rear. Here, the expertise of the psychiatric nurses and technicians of the OM team could be of great assistance in dealing with both problem and routine cases, as discussed earlier.   However, there was neither the need nor the resources to staff a 24 hour a day psychiatric ward this far forward; the needed expertise could be provided by one psychiatric nurse and two psychiatric technicians. Occupational therapy expertise was seen as valuable to organize and run the work and recreational activities, which are a major part of restoring the battle fatigued soldier's confidence. This lesson was demonstrated during World War I. The inclusion of occupational therapy in the combat mental health team was made official in the 1984 update of Army Regulation AR 40-216.

Implementing the Combat Stress Control Unit Concept

The Medical System Program Review approved the proposal to update the OM team into more mobile, modular, and multidisciplinary Combat Stress Control companies and detachments. The fielding plan authorized a great increase in the number of corps level CSC units and total personnel over the one active and six reserve OM teams in the current inventory. The organizational and operational concept paper was directed primarily at the NATO high intensity scenario, but also considered the use of CSC units in low intensity conflicts.   The TO&E development process eventually culminated in the detailed specifications for two types of CSC units, one smaller and one larger than the OM team.

The TO&Es for these two units were written in 1986 and revised in 1988 and passed their first Training and Doctrine Command (TRADOC) board proceeding in June 1989. They then waited in queue for the few hours of work needed to transfer them to a different computer format so they could be forwarded for staffing at the Department of Army and Major Commands. They were still in that queue in August 1990 when Saddam Hussein's Iraqi Army invaded Kuwait. Consequently, the Army went to war with what it had—the old OM team TO&E.

Deployment Status for Corps Level Mental Health (OM) Teams

This section provides an overview of the predeployment and mobilization situation for the three corps level mental health teams activated and deployed to the Gulf War. It records who and what were deployed to Saudi Arabia; it does not attempt to assign individual blame for problems that were experienced in the process.   As with the division mental health sections, the problems were systematic.

The 528th Medical Detachment, an Active Component OM Team. The 528th OM team was activated at Fort Benning in mid September. Its PROFIS officers were gathered from multiple posts. Several came from Fort Benning or the Eisenhower Medical Center and had been working together. Others had known individuals in the newly assembled unit from previous tours; some did not. The enlisted personnel were levied from across the country. They were sometimes picked by the personnel managers or the post commander because they were the most recent arrival or the most dispensable because of the position they occupied. They proved to be a good group, however.

There was a delay in designating the commander for the 528th. Initially, the PROFIS designated commander was to be replaced by a colonel in the Surgeon General's Office, who had more prior experience as a division psychiatrist. However, that colonel felt that he would be better used as the psychiatry consultant at Army Central Command Headquarters in Saudi Arabia. While that was being negotiated, most of the unit members were assembling at Fort Benning, without a commander. Finally, another psychiatrist colonel (at that time director of the Eisenhower Medical Center residency training program, and with strong prior experience as both division psychiatrist and division surgeon) was designated and arrived. As described in chapter 4, he did a superb job.

Even with the new commander's efforts, the 528th deployed at C3 status, the minimum acceptable for deployment overseas. It was short one psychiatrist (as a result of a medical condition diagnosed during the predeployment physical exam) and several key NCOs. It anticipated the new Combat Stress Control detachment TO&E by having an occupational therapy officer in the place of one social work officer (who was released on compassionate grounds), and an occupational therapy enlisted specialist instead of one behavioral science specialist. Its four pickup trucks, four-wheel-drive vehicles, and single two and a half-ton truck were in questionable repair, as a result of years of hard use is support of other missions. A suggestion to the Army's Forces Command Headquarters (FORSCOM) that the 528th be allowed to add a second two and a half-ton truck to more closely approach the greater carrying capability of the future CSC detachments was rejected out of hand—the argument being that any such effort to modify the weight and cube of the unit in midstream would be incompatible with the computer specified scheduling of the transport aircraft.

Other Reserve OM Teams Deployed to the Gulf War. In August 1990, two U.S. Army Reserve OM teams were placed on the classified Time-Phased Force Deployment List for deployment to Saudi Arabia. The units themselves were not notified and were not scheduled to fly until about Christmas. The two units were from the East Coast (the 383rd in Boston and the 531st in Baltimore). They may have been picked because they had prior European or Rapid Deployment Force contingency missions assigned to them. The two units which were initially (and secretly) selected were not the most ready by virtue of their recent training.

The 383rd (Boston) was well motivated to deploy but had little field experience and an odd personnel mix (overstrength in psychiatric nurses, but lacking in psychiatrists and other positions). The 531st (Baltimore) had been a proud Rapid Deployment Force unit until the mid-1980s. It had trained under the 44th Medical Brigade at Fort Bragg in 1984 and 1985 and been declared combat-ready. It had performed very well at a major field exercise at Camp Shelby, Mississippi, in June 1986, where its teams had functioned in the widely dispersed and mobile mode called for in the evolving CSC doctrine. Since then, however, it had suffered from an absence of consistent leadership (eventually not having a psychiatrist or physician commander). The result had been internal dissension within and between the mental health disciplines and the officer/NCO structure. This had been evident during another major field exercise at Camp Shelby in 1989.

The Friday before Thanksgiving, the 531st (Baltimore) and the 467th (Madison, Wisconsin) were alerted to mobilize the day before Thanksgiving and to be at their mobilization site the Saturday after Thanksgiving. They would have ten days to load and be ready on the airfield to deploy.

This came as a surprise—especially the selection of the 467th in place of the 383rd from Boston. The Wisconsin team was the least field experienced team of all the six reserve OM teams; it had trained to be a CONUS hospital augmentation unit (although one social work officer and several noncommissioned officers had come on their own to the big medical field training exercises where the combat stress control doctrine had been tested). It was ironic and perhaps fated that the author had been invited to Madison, Wisconsin, the last weekend in July 1990 to conduct a workshop on combat stress for the 467th. The reception had been cordial, but the reaction of most of the unit members seemed to have been that this was all academic. With the Soviet Union reforming, there was not even that chance that they might be deployed outside the United States to provide combat stress control. Reportedly, the Forces Command decision of which team to send to the Persian Gulf was made purely and objectively from the Unit Status Reports (USR). If so, the USR statements of personnel and equipment on hand failed to record the relevant data or were themselves miscompleted.

The 531st from Baltimore had a Medical Corps commander, but he was a nuclear medicine physician, not a psychiatrist. He was exempted from having to deploy. There was no psychiatrist who had drilled with the unit, but three were identified by the First Army Augmentation Detachment (FAAD) or National Augmentation Detachment (NAD) computer files as belonging to it.

The senior one (a lieutenant colonel) was a psychiatrist for the State Department who had experience in the Middle East and Central America. However, with the short notice call up, he could not be notified because he was sailing his ketch solo across the Atlantic to Spain. When finally contacted, he had to attend the second of the one week crash Officer Basic Courses (OBC) given at Fort Sam Houston, San Antonio. This course filled a statutory requirement before any officer could be deployed overseas. This psychiatrist did eventually catch up to the unit in Saudi Arabia, but he did not take over command.

The second ranking psychiatrist, also a lieutenant colonel, had 11 years of active duty experience, but most as a child psychiatrist in Army hospitals. He had been in private and academic practice since leaving the Army. He had to come for the first pre Christmas short Officer Basic Course, and he ate his first Meal Ready to Eat (MRE) during the course. As a result, he arrived at the mobilization site only days before the unit's departure and was unable to complete the required qualification in time. It took him several weeks to catch up to the unit in Saudi to assume command.

Meanwhile, acting command had fallen to the third reserve psychiatrist, a major (promotable) but not yet close to his promotion date. He had strong active duty experience, notably as a member of the 7th Medical Command's Stress Management Team in Heidelberg, Germany. He had been involved in several crisis hostage situations, which had taken him as far as Pakistan. Now he found himself in an extremely chaotic command situation in a unit whose internal politics were already disruptive, with little time to prepare for deployment to a potentially lethal combat zone.

The only other psychiatrist which the computer based NAD system could produce to deploy with the 531st was a mid-fifties female psychiatrist who was cross-leveled from a General Hospital in Florida. Although she had been in the Reserves at least 8 years and was a major, she had always been in hospital units which would be deployed to a communications zone. She was at this time semiretired for health reasons after a career in the New York City psychiatric emergency hospitalization field, but she was still deployable and went. While one might have unbounded admiration for her heroism, it is only fair to say that she did not have the field experience or the stamina which the CSC concept had envisioned as necessary for working well forward with combat arms divisions and brigades. (In Saudi, she switched positions with a younger psychiatrist from an Evacuation Hospital.) The psychologist for the 531st also was a Reservist cross leveled from a Pennsylvania unit. She did not arrive in time to deploy with the 531st and had to catch up with the unit in Saudi Arabia.

Having deployed under these adverse circumstances in the first week of December, it is hardly surprising that the 531st had difficulty establishing unit cohesion in the theater.

The 467th from Madison also had a difficult deployment. The commander, a 60-year-old Filipino American psychiatrist, was in the Philippines on compassionate grounds because of an ill parent. She was eligible but declined mandatory retirement, and she elected to lead her unit to war. Again, one can admire her personal courage and loyalty to her unit without seeing her as the ideal commander for a forward deploying combat stress control unit (because of her lack of military and field experience and credibility with the combat arms). The other drilling psychiatrist failed to report for deployment, citing medical problems.

To fill the four missing psychiatrist positions, the NAD called up another over-60 female psychiatrist from a reserve general hospital in Florida (whose mission had been to reinforce a communications zone, not to deploy into the Combat Zone). She showed remarkably good grace and positive attitude when reporting to the bitter cold of Fort McCoy, after having been uncivilly threatened with prosecution by the officials who had contacted her by phone because she did not report on time (they had been unable to contact her while she was away from home visiting her grandchildren). Fortunately, the 467th's mission in Saudi Arabia allowed her to remain with a small part of the unit to provide the mental health support for theater level units in Riyadh, Saudi Arabia. Even in this role, at her age she was a true Gulf War heroine.

A more doctrinally apt choice for the third psychiatrist to deploy with the 467th was a Pakistani American psychiatrist from California sent by the NAD. He had attended the regular Officer Basic Course a year or two before, but for some reason he was sent to the pre-Christmas short OBC at San Antonio, too. Fortunately, he was just barely able to reach Fort McCoy, Wisconsin, complete deployment qualification requirements and deploy with the unit. The 467th was still short two psychiatrists and the clinical psychologist when it deployed the first week in December. Like the other two OM teams, it was deployed at the minimally acceptable C3 status.

CONCLUSION

In January 1991, as the air campaign began, all division level mental health sections were in place, and no additional corps level stress control units beyond the 528th, 531st, and 467th were programmed to deploy. Official casualty projections for wounded in action were high, based on the possibility of having to fight determined Iraqi veterans in their well prepared defensive positions in a chemical and perhaps biological environment. Assuming the historically validated ratios of battle fatigue casualties to wounded in action (BFC:WIA) of 1:5, 1:3, or even 1:2 (in the chemical scenario), it was clear that three understrength corps level OM teams would not be adequate.

After extensive staff work by the acting Consultant for Neuropsychiatry to the Army Surgeon General, the Surgeon General and the Army's Deputy Chief of Staff for Personnel jointly sent a message to the Commander of Army Central Command. The message stated that the consensus of Army medical opinion from evolving doctrine was that all seven available active and reserve psychiatric detachments (OM teams) should be in theater. It suggested that consideration be given to bringing over the remaining teams.

As it happened, the successful ground campaign was waged before any action was taken on the message. The division mental health sections and the three OM teams, deployed far forward, proved sufficient to manage the small number of stress casualties seen during and immediately after the victory. That number was fully consistent with projections for a short and victorious campaign and with the small number of U.S. personnel killed and wounded. It was noted in the subsequent lessons-learned process that the forward deployment of most of the OM team assets did mean that there were not sufficient CSC resources in the corps rear and echelon above corps to fully cover the combat stress threat generated by the Scud missiles. It is also becoming increasingly evident that more CSC resources in theater could have been used in demobilization and prehomecoming debriefings, to minimize posttraumatic or deployment distress.

This is jumping ahead. With this introduction to what should have been available for U.S. Army deployment to Saudi Arabia under the old and the new (but not yet fielded) TO&Es, and what actually was deployed, it is time to learn what these individuals and their units actually did.

2

Army Mental Health Units in the Theater of Operations: An Overview of the Gulf War

James A. Martin and Joe G. Fagan

INTRODUCTION

This chapter examines the nature and operations of U.S. Army mental health units deployed to Southwest Asia (SWA) during the Gulf War. It describes the U.S. Army's efforts to establish mental health resources in the theater of operations capable of sustaining soldiers in a physically, psychologically, and socially hostile environment, and to respond to the psychiatric requirements of an army about to engage in what was expected to be the largest and most violent land based conflict since World War II.

MENTAL HEALTH ISSUES

The term "fog of battle" refers to the confusion and indecision that occurs during combat operations. In reviewing the preliminary senior level headquarters planning for mental health support for the Gulf War, it is apparent that the fog of battle can occur before any shots are fired. Initially the perception among senior medical planners was that the deployment of troops from the Army's rapid reaction force, the 82nd Airborne Division, was primarily a show of force rather than the first step in a major deployment of American forces. The prevailing view in Washington was that Iraq would back down in the face of the presence of the U.S. Forces and the outrage of world opinion. The worst-case scenario was thought to be a brief battle with few physical and/or psychiatric casualties and with U.S. airpower occupying a dominant role. Planning for combat stress reaction (CSR) in large numbers was essentially on the back burner, although past experience with extended training and peacekeeping deployments in the Middle East had demonstrated the need for mental health support.

When the troops from the 82nd Airborne Division prepared to deploy to Saudi Arabia, there was optimism in the Army Surgeon General's Office in Washington that the 82nd would deploy their division mental health team and that this would be a sufficient mental health response. The expectation that the 82nd would include mental health personnel on their deployment manifest was based on the established need for garrison-type mental health services in this remote environment rather than any expectation that there would be significant ground combat with corresponding numbers of combat stress casualties.

As events began to unfold and more forces were committed to SWA, the primary mental health concern among Army medical planners in Washington was the obvious stress associated with the extremely hostile and demanding physical, social, and psychological environment in the SWA theater of operations. No one, from the senior generals in Washington to the privates in the desert, knew how long this deployment would last.

The majority of the men and women in this force were married (while many others were single parents or had significant extended family responsibilities). Many of these soldiers and their families, especially reserve and national guard members, were admittedly not prepared for a lengthy, open ended separation from home and family. At the same time, national and local news programs back home began highlighting the personal and family stressors associated with this deployment. Live television provided a look at some of the hardships of desert life for soldiers (especially women trying to deal with the restrictions of a Moslem culture), examined the personal sacrifices and hardships for many of those deployed (especially reservists whose employment and income was affected by their call up), and, through gripping interviews and stories, highlighted the economic and social stress experienced by some families at home.

Once it was clear to the Army's senior medical leaders that an offensive war was possible, if not inevitable, the focus of medical planning shifted to the possibility, if not probability, of large numbers of combat casualties, including combat stress reactions (also referred to in Army literature as battle fatigue casualties). There was a general expectation that a land war in the desert would be extremely lethal and possibly involve the use of chemical and biological weapons. Many credible sources predicted large numbers of dead and wounded and enormous numbers of combat stress casualties (a ratio of one stress casualty for every three combat deaths was the expected norm, with higher ratios in the event of especially intense combat situations).

Under these circumstances, there was a clear public message that a repeat of the Vietnam War scenario, in which thousands of veterans returned with posttraumatic stress disorder (PTSD), would be unacceptable. Prevention and early treatment of combat stress reactions became a medical priority. Even well-informed combat leaders, who recognized that their cohesive, well-led, well-trained, and well-equipped units, operating in the offense, would be buffeted from what otherwise might be overwhelming stress, felt a need for additional preparation; these leaders often requested last minute combat stress training for their soldiers.

This chapter describes the activities of Army mental health units in SWA during the build up and the sustainment period leading up to the start of the air and ground war. There were a number of deficiencies in the selection and preparation of mental health personnel and units deployed to SWA (Martin, 1992), as well as problems in the timing and adequacy of the mental health resources deployed to SWA (Martin and Cline, 1992). Regardless of these deficiencies, some well-trained, flexible, and creative mental health professionals were able to establish a safety net believed capable of preventing a hemorrhage of combat stress casualties from SWA. Fortunately, because of the nature of the ground war (a five-day, extremely successful, fast-paced, single ground offensive with only a small number of American dead or wounded, and the absence of chemical and biological weapons), this mental health safety net was never really tested.

ARMY MENTAL HEALTH UNITS

This section describes Army combat mental health resources and provides background information on problems encountered in fielding mental health units for the Gulf War deployment. It discusses the Saudi Arabian deployment and preparation for a ground offensive into Iraq. Issues at each level of the combat mental health system are covered, as well as strategic planning for the ground combat.

Division Mental Health Teams

The first Army mental health personnel in theater were members of the division mental health teams from the four divisions of the XVIII Corps that arrived in Saudi Arabia between August and October 1991. A typical division mental health team consists of three officers—a psychiatrist, psychologist, social worker—and five to seven enlisted behavioral science specialists. In a deployed environment, a division mental health team's primary role includes unit consultation, screening evaluations, and limited brief treatment. These tasks require a mental health team that is well trained, is experienced in field operations, and has sufficient mobility to operate in a division's widely dispersed operational environment. As described elsewhere (Martin, 1992), few of these division mental health teams possessed these attributes or assets when they arrived in SWA. The tasks were made more difficult because most of these Army divisions were deployed at 20 percent overstrength in anticipation of possible combat losses. They were augmented with additional combat support units, making these division task forces 20 to 30 percent larger than their normal peacetime garrison configuration.

For most of these division mental health teams, the Gulf War learning curve was steep.   The task of obtaining adequate equipment, especially tactical vehicles, was extremely frustrating.   This was especially true for VII Corps division mental health teams, which did not arrive in SWA until December. Without vehicles, it was nearly impossible for these mental health teams to reach widely dispersed divisional units to provide consultation and combat stress training.

By the start of the ground war in late February 1991, most division mental health teams had obtained some transportation assets and had reached an acceptable readiness level.   They were just beginning to provide critical mental health training and consultation services.   In most cases, however, these tasks and the potential confrontation with large numbers of combat stress casualties were still well beyond their team's inherent operational capabilities.

The situation was particularly difficult for the three division mental health teams that deployed in January 1991 as part of VII Corps (two from Europe and one from the United States).   These teams had many of the same training deficiencies and equipment problems as the XVIII Corps teams, compounded by even greater predeployment staffing problems.   Despite these deficiencies, these teams demonstrated heroic efforts to reach an acceptable readiness status before the start of the ground war.

There were clearly some significant holes in unit level mental health coverage for combat forces deployed throughout the theater of operations.   In fact, a number of front line Army combat units, including an armored Cavalry regiment and a separate armored brigade, arrived in Saudi Arabia without organic mental health support.

Combat Field Hospitals

By September 15, 1990, three Army hospitals were operating in SWA. By November 30, this number had reached eight. On January 15, 1991, forty-one hospitals were in the field, and at the start of the ground war on February 24, 1991, forty-four Army hospitals were operating in SWA. These hospital units included eight Mobile Army Surgical Hospitals (MASH), nine Combat Support Hospitals (CSH), twenty-two Evacuation Hospitals (EVAC), one Station Hospital, three Field Hospitals, and one General Hospital. Sixteen of these hospitals were from the Army's active component, and twenty eight were Reserve Component hospitals. Twelve hospitals supported XVIII Corps, fifteen supported V Corps, and the rest were assigned as theater level assets.

Many of these hospitals had staff members with some mental health training, especially Reserve Component units with individuals who had civilian jobs as social workers, school counselors, or psychiatric nurses. In particular, many reserve hospitals had staffed a variety of their difficult to fill medical and surgical nursing positions with available psychiatric nurses. The Evacuation, Field, and General Hospitals all had an organic mental health section and a specific inpatient psychiatric mission. Unfortunately, like the division mental health teams, many of those Evacuation Hospitals had little or no field experience, and there were a variety of specialty mismatches among their professional personnel. On the positive side, a number of these Evacuation Hospitals were able to provide notable mental health services during the sustainment period before the ground war began. They were often the only source of mental health services that units could find as forces began movement up to the Iraqi border in preparation for the ground offensive. For logistical reasons, most of these hospitals were located on main supply routes and were relatively easy to locate. On the negative side, one of these Evacuation Hospitals, inadequately and improperly staffed and located near a major airfield, became the source of the majority of the Desert Shield (sustainment period) psychiatric evacuations from SWA.

OM Teams

Chapter 4 provides a detailed description of the organization, mission, and deployment of the corps level mental health teams deployed to SWA. In the simplest sense, these 48 plus-member mental health units were designed to operate behind and in support of division mental health teams. Ideally, they provide limited holding capacity (80 to 100 cots) for combat stress reaction casualties evacuated from division level care. They are also designed to provide brief treatment for casualties coming from nondivisional units operating in their vicinity. These units were expected to provide enough mental health personnel to augment and support divisional mental health teams during and immediately after combat.

When the Gulf War began, the Army was already involved in a lengthy and delayed conversion of the OM team concept to a new organization (combat stress control company or CSCC) being developed under the Army Medical Department's future combat organization—a plan called Medical Force 2000. A number of these CSCCs actually existed in the Reserve Component, and a few had even conducted limited field training. Unfortunately, the Office of the Army Surgeon General was not able to override the Army's preexisting deployment plan, and OM teams were deployed rather than CSCCs. This resulted in the deployment of one Active Component OM team (this team existed on paper but was not organized, equipped, or trained) and the call up and deployment of two existing Reserve Component OM teams (which, because of an inadequate readiness reporting system, were, at least on paper, listed as ready for deployment while in fact these teams were improperly staffed, ill equipped, and untrained).

In addition to the personnel, training, and equipment deficiencies found in these three OM Teams (see the details in Chapters 4 and 15) the delays in actual call up and deployment, and the deficiency in the total number of teams deployed, caused grave concern for Army mental health leaders. Based on Army doctrine, including the size of the force deployed in SWA and the potential lethality of the conflict, a minimum of seven of these mental health teams were required. Instead, three untrained and ill equipped OM teams were sent to the combat zone, all later than required (one in late October and the other two in December). Mental health leaders saw all of this as a recipe for disaster in light of the perceived potential for significant battle fatigue casualties. In fact, the Army's Academy of Health Science computer simulations predicted 1400 battle fatigue casualties per week in the expected SWA ground combat. With adequate mental health staffing in SWA, these computer models suggested that 1190 soldiers could be expected to return to duty. With the proposed staffing, fewer than 560 soldiers would actually be returned to duty. This set the stage for unnecessary evacuations and high rates of prolonged mental dysfunction and disability. Offsetting this fear was the general recognition that good leadership, small unit cohesion, realistic training, and state of the art equipment in the active component force would help reduce overall battle fatigue casualties.

Through early December 1990, in-theater mental health efforts focused primarily on equipping and training these teams and initiating a variety of outreach activities at corps and theater levels, as well as, some initial liaison with the division mental health teams. The arrival of the first (Active Component) OM team did dramatically reduce the number of psychiatric evacuations out of the theater. By operating in the same area as the hospitals and airfields in the rear (gateways out of the theater of operations), these mental health personnel had the opportunity to serve as effective gatekeepers, intervening in a variety of situations where return to duty was possible.

THE THEATER PSYCHIATRIC CONSULTANT

During an early October 1990 visit to Saudi Arabia by a Headquarters Department of the Army team studying stress issues, the theater surgeon identified his need for a senior staff psychiatrist (referred to here as the theater psychiatry consultant) and a preventive medicine officer. The theater surgeon clearly articulated mental health issues and preventive medicine concerns as critical threats to the Army's ability to sustain forces for a prolonged period in the hostile SWA environment. At the Pentagon, there was an initial belief that the psychiatrist serving as the commander of the Active Component OM team would be able to function in both the role of OM Team unit commander, as well as the theater psychiatry consultant (this can be seen as part of the same fog of battle described earlier). Once on the ground in Saudi Arabia, the OM team commander quickly recognized that this dual hat responsibility would not work. Besides the enormous task of completing the readiness requirements for his OM team, the great distances and lack of adequate communications made it impossible to function adequately in both roles. The recognition of this reality resulted in the deployment of a second senior psychiatrist to perform the function of the Army theater psychiatry consultant.

It is worth noting that the Army theater surgeon requested a preventive medicine consultant and a psychiatry consultant months before requesting a medicine consultant and a surgical consultant. The medicine and surgical consultants arrived in Saudi Arabia after the fundamental decisions with regard to the deployment of medical and surgical assets had already been made. Their earlier input would have been helpful. Fortunately, the same was not true for mental health planning.

The Army theater psychiatric consultant who deployed to Saudi Arabia in early November 1990 was air evacuated out of the theater for medical treatment after being there for less than a week. During this brief period, he advised the Army theater surgeon that the number of anticipated combat stress reactions, in accordance with accepted doctrine, would grossly overwhelm the existing theater mental health capability. Current doctrine indicated that the shortfall of mental health resources at that point was about 60 percent. The consultant's evacuation out of theater put this assessment on hold until his replacement arrived. In the United States, however, there was very little urgency with regard to the replacement of the theater psychiatric consultant. It appears in retrospect that the initial assessment of mental health needs was thought to be of such magnitude that it lacked credibility. For whatever reason, the new Army theater psychiatry consultant did not deploy to Saudi Arabia until early December 1990. Considerable planning time was lost in this process, along with the opportunity to obtain additional mental health personnel to meet theater combat stress control requirements.

The new psychiatry consultant functioned as one of a number of staff officers and senior advisors to the Army's theater surgeon. In this capacity, he had the opportunity to influence a number of important decisions and policies with direct and indirect impacts on mental health in the SWA theater of operations. A very important accomplishment was the redistribution of mental health assets in the corps and theater mental health units in preparation for the start of the ground offensive. This redistribution allowed a reconfiguration that took into consideration the projected combat scenario, as well as the skills and training of various OM team and hospital unit members. The psychiatry consultant's frequent presence in the field significantly enhanced the morale of theater and corps mental health personnel. This direct contact was the Consultant's primary source of up-to-date information from the field. While the consultant could pick up a Headquarters office phone and talk directly to the United States, he had no reliable telephone or radio link to any of the corps or theater mental health teams or hospitals. For information, he had to make personal contact on the ground.

At the end of the ground war, the consultant prepared combat stress debriefing guidance that was issued by the theater Army commander. Unfortunately, the guidance was late and not mandatory. As a result, many units did not comply with it. The urge for demobilization was so strong throughout the force, including most mental health personnel, that any effort that even hinted at the potential to extend their time in Saudi Arabia was extremely unpopular. Hospitals were packed up as soon as permission was granted in order to not be caught in Saudi Arabia with beds filled with patients.

THE WALTER REED ARMY INSTITUTE OF RESEARCH HUMAN DIMENSION STRESS TEAM

Early in the Gulf War deployment, a team of social scientists from the Walter Reed Army Institute of Research (WRAIR) deployed to Saudi Arabia to assess the stress associated with sustaining soldiers in this hostile environment. Their assessment was to be used by Army leaders to help determine a rotational policy for what appeared to be an open ended commitment of military forces in SWA. Once soldiers heard the Secretary of Defense's announcement that there would be no rotations and that their way home was through Iraq, the soldiers shifted their focus. There clear objective was the defeat of the Iraqi Army. At this point, additional WRAIR stress teams collected interview and survey data from soldiers to help senior leaders devise ways to reduce stress during the necessarily prolonged build up phase leading to the start of the actual ground war.

One of these teams (a senior psychiatrist and social worker) operated in the VII Corps area during the build up phase, collecting observational and survey data in divisional units. The team also provided combat stress training and consultation support to division and corps mental health personnel. With their own transportation (a rental vehicle) and operating as an asset of the theater psychiatry consultant, they were an extension of his efforts and a source of valuable information on mental health unit readiness and personnel requirements and deployment of assets across the corps.

Just prior to the start of the ground war, these officers combined with another psychiatrist and a sergeant from the VII Corps OM team and formed a mental health team for one of the Armored Cavalry Regiments set to lead the ground offensive. Operating out of and with support from the Cavalry Regiment's medical troop, this mental health team was able to ride circuit throughout the regiment and its many recently attached combat and combat support units. These precombat consultations with front-line medical personnel and unit chaplains, as well as visits with many of the regiment's senior officers and NCOs, were used to reinforce basic battle fatigue prevention and treatment principles and to introduce the concept of stress debriefings.

These contacts proved invaluable immediately after combat. They facilitated team access to a number of regimental units for critical incident debriefings after incidents of friendly fire and other combat related deaths and injuries (Chapter 9 for a detailed description). These critical incident debriefings helped soldiers realistically confront the trauma of combat and make sense out of their normal reaction to an often overwhelming psychological experience. The critical incident stress debriefing helped soldiers talk through their experience, clarify misconceptions, and set the stage for open conversation among peers and leaders that provided a source of tremendous interpersonal support.

Based on the experiences and accomplishments of this mental health team, it is clear that units like armored Cavalry regiments require organic mental health resources whenever they deploy into combat. It is also clear that the assignment of senior, experienced mental health officers in far forward locations provides the opportunity for important mental health interventions.

PREPARING FOR COMBAT OPERATIONS

As the inevitable ground war approached, available mental health resources consisted of the divisional mental health teams, OM teams, limited psychiatric resources in the Evacuation Hospitals, and a Psychiatric Inpatient Unit in the one Theater General Hospital. As noted earlier, these mental health resources were not adequately sized, structured, trained, or equipped for the combat tasks anticipated in any major ground offensive. The total combat stress reaction holding capacity was less than 30 cots in each division mental health team, 75 cots for the three OM teams, no psychiatric beds in the Evacuation Hospitals, and only one 50-bed psychiatric unit in the General Hospital. These limited resources would need to manage the total combat stress reactions of an Army force of over 300,000 soldiers posed for what was anticipated to be the most intense and violent desert armor battle in military history.

Early predictions of combat stress reactions were about 150 per day per corps, or about 300 total per day in the theater of operations. However, it is necessary to note that these estimates were based on the classified projections for total wounded and/or killed in action. They did not reflect the unequal distribution of combat stress reactions throughout the course of the predicted ground war. Typically, the bulk of combat stress reactions occur in the beginning of a war. For purposes of attempting to project more accurately the potential surge of combat stress reactions in the first few days of this war, an estimate was made based on military studies of previous conflicts. This demonstrated a linear decline in combat stress reactions over the first week of exposure to combat, followed by a relatively stable rate for the next three weeks, followed by another rapid increase presumably secondary to combat related physiological fatigue.

Using this model for guidance, the estimates for combat stress reactions over the initial 30-day time frame were redistributed, with 40 percent of the combat stress reactions predicted to occur in the first week of combat. During that first week, this model predicted a linear decline over each of the first seven days of combat. This model resulted in a better illustration of the tasks facing the mental health providers in managing combat stress reactions. This resulted in an estimate of 900 combat stress reactions for day 1 with a decline each day of 50 until a steady state of 140 per day was reached at the end of the first week. Under these circumstances, it was obvious that the Army mental health resources in the Saudi Arabian theater of operations were inadequate in simple numbers (by Army doctrine the shortfall was about 170 mental health providers, or about 60 percent of the minimum personnel requirements and about an 80 percent shortfall in unit equipment). The doctrinal organization of these mental health units did not permit even their inadequate numbers from being deployed in an effective manner. This exacerbated the overall shortfall in mental health resources.

The official threat assessment, with associated casualty estimates, clearly demonstrated that the combat stress reactions would almost immediately overwhelm the existing mental health system. This would naturally lead to the rapid medical evacuation of combat stress reactions out of the theater of operations beginning on the second day of ground combat. This was clearly not in the best interests of the soldiers being evacuated in terms of the potential for long-term psychiatric morbidity. It was also not in the best interests of their commanders, who stood to lose significant numbers of soldiers unnecessarily. The situation was clearly unacceptable.

A decision was made by the theater psychiatric consultant in late December 1990 to concentrate combat stress control efforts on maximizing the effectiveness of existing resources rather than continuing futile efforts to obtain additional resources. Overall military air-and sea-lift capability was stretched to its limits such that strict guidance was issued by the theater Headquarters as to what kind of unit substitutions could be made for units still to be deployed to Saudi Arabia. In regard to mental health units, it meant that to add another OM team, a complete hospital would have to be deleted from the list of units yet to be deployed. This was not likely to happen because of increasing concern among medical planners about the potential of large numbers of combat trauma casualties.

To expeditiously explore the ramifications of the various options available given these constrained resources and to select the best possible course of action, a series of mathematical models were developed to simulate the effectiveness of varying approaches to the task at hand. The primary constraint was the limit on mental health resources: people, vehicles, and communication equipment. All were inadequate; additional resources were not anticipated until well after the planned ground war was underway.

The combat mental health support plan for the upcoming ground war had to be understandable by both medical and line commanders. It also had to have face validity with the mental health providers while operating within their existing resource constraints. This plan had to be sufficiently generalizable for the theater as a whole so that pressure could be brought to bear on commanders to support the plan, yet the plan had to be flexible enough that individual mental health units could adapt it to their particular requirements while not allowing some commanders to use the flexibility as an excuse to support the mental health plan minimally.

In the development of conceptual models for the deployment of theater mental health resources, considerable weight was given to efforts to replicate the combat stress control (CSC) unit strategies that were under development as part of future Army doctrine. It was not an easy transition to the CSC model. There was the 40 percent shortfall in personnel and 80 percent shortfall in equipment to contend with, along with a command structure that was initially incompatible with the implementation of the new doctrine.

Several assumptions were made in the modeling process. The most important was the assumption of a 1:4 ratio of combat stress reactions to wounded in action and that, with appropriate management, a return-to-duty rate of 30 percent could be expected every 24 hours at each echelon of care. This represents an approximate 90 percent return to duty rate within 72 hours of treatment. This model predicted that there would be about 250 combat stress reactions per day for the first week of combat (although other models suggested that there would be an initial peak and then a subsequent decline in combat stress casualties across an initial period of conflict). Each corps was considered separately, as their tactical missions were different and casualties were projected to be higher for VII Corps because of its expected direct assault on dug-in, well-defended enemy forces. Given the limited capacity of the Iraqi Army to project their forces into the rear areas of the U.S. forces, it was also assumed that the great majority of combat stress reactions would develop within the forward divisional areas of operation, and therefore the generation of combat stress reactions could be funneled though division mental health personnel operating at forward brigade clearing stations.

The models demonstrated that, at a minimum, each divisional mental health section operating at the brigade clearing stations would need at least 40 combat casualty cots, that each OM team in support of a corps would need 120 combat casualty cots, and that each Evacuation Hospital would need 20 psychiatric beds if combat stress reactions were to be held in theater rather than evacuated to Europe and then on to the United States. These estimates were the absolute minimum and assumed optimum functioning of the entire evacuation and treatment system.

It was clear that any strategy for managing combat stress reactions needed to be sustainable for at least one week. Operational plans called for the bulk of the ground combat to be over by the end of the first week. Certainly, the majority of the combat stress reactions would occur within the first week. To manage the number and rate of these casualties, it would be necessary to generate a total of 700 to 800 cots/hospital beds in theater dedicated to combat stress reactions.

Next, it was necessary to determine the feasibility and limitations at each echelon of care and to maximize their capability. This process required balancing personnel, equipment, and transportation, as each could be a rate limiting factor. It became obvious that a mental health officer's value, as measured in ability to treat and return to duty combat stress reactions, increased proportionately to his or her proximity to the front and vice versa. Thus, priority was given to shifting mental health treatment capability to the front, as this was the most cost-effective use of limited resources. Conceptually this meant maximizing the effort to replicate doctrinally based division mental health team and OM team restoration functions (providing a few hours to a few days of brief supportive treatment) in the divisional areas of operation by limiting the capability for corps-and theater level reconstitution and imposing even more significant limitations for retraining (both reconstitution and retraining are focused on providing for longer, more involved treatment interventions for the most severe combat stress reactions). restoration would be primarily the responsibility of the OM teams collocated with the forward Mobile Army Surgical Hospital (MASH) and Combat Support Hospitals (CSH), while the Evacuation (EVAC) Hospitals, because of their rather austere settings and their own location far forward in this scenario, were to be utilized for reconstitution. Only one reconditioning unit was set up at a major staging area located at a military base in northeast Saudi Arabia. This plan would achieve about 80 percent of the goal for the restoration mission, about 20 percent of the reconstitution mission, and a negligible retraining mission. By definition, this also meant a significant shortfall for mental health services for the rear echelon troops.

All of the potential resources for this plan for the management of combat stress reactions belonged to separate senior commanders. It was necessary to negotiate separately with each commander. Medical policy guidance was the responsibility of the Army theater surgeon but implementation was the purview of each unit/facility commander.

The operational model selected differed from that outlined for doctrinally based combat stress control units in several important ways. Of necessity, it was less ambitious in scope due to limited resources. It abandoned the doctrinal concept of a dual evacuation chain with combat stress reactions isolated from all other medical/surgical cases. Resource constraints in terms of communications, transportation, and the capacity of many mental health units to be self-sustaining would not allow for dual evacuations. The model did retain the emphasis on the restoration teams (brief far-forward intervention) while significantly reducing the reconstitution units and essentially eliminating retraining units (rear area, more intensive interventions).

In December 1991, the senior mental health officers on the ground in SWA confronted the reality of available mental health resources and implemented the measures just described to reconfigure assets in order to meet what they considered a realistic appraisal of the threat (a 1:3 combat stress reactions to wounded in action ratio, peaking in the first seven days and then declining to produce an average of as many as 150 combat stress reactions per corps per day over the first 30 days of ground combat). In addition, it was clear that the nature of the proposed ground offensive (a fast-moving assault) would result in an abandonment of the basic principle of using only ground evacuation for battle fatigue casualties. Mental health personnel had to expect that all casualties would be moved by air, regardless of their condition, and that local (unit level) treatment facilities would often be bypassed as patients were flown to rear area hospitals.

The next step in preparing for the expected ground offensive was to cross level the three OM teams by shifting personnel and vehicles from the OM team designated to support the echelons above corps to the teams supporting each of the two corps. This allowed these corps level units to reconfigure from one treatment team and three consultation teams into four treatment teams and a headquarters section. Each of these four- to six-person treatment teams would be able to provide a 20 cot holding capability. The plan called for these teams to collocate with the forward-deployed MASHs and CSHs and provide area mental health support. While this provided an effective structure and placement, there was still recognition that holding capability was less than sufficient for the expected need.

A third step was to establish a 20-bed minimal care holding capability at each EVAC Hospital for battle fatigue casualties. This would provide a necessary back up for the corps OM teams. By the start of the ground war, this plan was accomplished.

The final step was to reconfigure the remaining assets from the theater level OM team and to establish a reconditioning unit capable of holding combat stress reactions in the theater for at least 14 days. This unit would be located at the airhead, receiving corps level evacuees in order to create a safety-net to prevent unnecessary evacuation out of the theater. It was believed that if these soldiers could be retained in the theater for this period, there would be considerable opportunity to return these soldiers to their units once the fighting stopped. This would allow the possibility of reintegrating these soldiers with their peers so they would not experience the isolation and perceived rejection that often follows an evacuation out of the combat theater. Establishing this reconditioning unit required additional personnel and time. Additional mental health personnel arrived from the United States just prior to the start of the ground offensive, and the reconditioning unit was put in place. Unfortunately, there was not sufficient time to prepare this unit adequately for its role or to integrate it into the area support medical care system.

SUMMARY

This chapter has examined the structure and operation of U.S. Army mental health personnel deployed to SWA during the Gulf War. It describes efforts to establish mental health resources capable of responding to the psychiatric requirements of what was expected to be the largest and most violent land based conflict since World War II. It is clear that division based mental health teams were not adequately staffed, equipped, or trained at the time of deployment for this type of combat operation. Corps level mental health units were even less prepared. The eventual presence of a senior mental health officer in the theater and the enormous amount of effort in the field resulted in the establishment of a mental health plan that provided a safety-net believed capable of stemming what could have been a flood of stress casualties. Fortunately, the extremely effective U.S. led five week air assault followed by the decisive ground assault into Iraq negated the use of chemical or biological weapons, and there were very few American casualties. The nature of this war and its very brief duration limited the number of American (and Coalition Forces) combat stress casualties.

While there were very few immediate combat stress casualties, it is still unclear how many individuals had an extreme stress experience sufficient to produce a posttraumatic stress response. Among these were soldiers involved in incidents of friendly fire and soldiers whose duties brought them into direct contact with the dead. It is also unclear how many soldiers experienced or will someday experience mental health consequences from the persistent physical, psychological, and social stress in the pre-and post-Gulf War environment and whose separation from home and family resulted in prolonged relationship problems. It is clear that the mental health units deployed to SWA were only marginally able to provide in theater mental health services and were not prepared to provide postcombat debriefing services. While there were a few cases of highly successful unit debriefings, this is an area of responsibility that needs to be emphasized in the mission and training of combat stress control units.

It is important to end by noting that most mental health personnel were able to rise above the many organizational deficiencies and, from the perspective of the individual clinician, they accomplished the mission.

3

Psychiatric Services in the Evacuation Zone: A View from the U.S. Army Psychiatric Consultant for U.S. Forces in Europe

William R. Cline

INTRODUCTION

This chapter has two purposes: first, to describe for future planners the range of complex issues needing attention when psychiatric support to a war effort is being designed as part of a greater medical system; second, to give the perspective of the psychiatric consultant for the U.S. Army 7th Medical Command (Europe).

For 7th Medical Command (MEDCOM), the Gulf War involved the massive deployment of medical soldiers from American forces in Europe to Southwest Asia (SWA) in anticipation of overwhelming numbers of casualties. It also meant coping with a workload associated with the peacetime medical requirements of remaining forces and military family members in Europe. Finally, 7th MEDCOM had to modify existing procedures and programs in its 11 hospitals in order to prepare to treat the anticipated Gulf War casualties.

Medical forces in general and psychiatric forces in particular in Europe were not ready for a "come as you are" war when the conflict in the Gulf began. We were fortunate that many weeks passed from the start of the air war phase of the Gulf War to the start of actual ground combat. Because of adequate time for training, reorganization, and receipt of reinforcements, psychiatry and the allied mental health professions in Europe eventually felt as prepared as possible for the worst-case war.

For at least 10 years before the war, there was no psychiatric annex to the medical "go to war" plans maintained at Headquarters (HQ) 7th MEDCOM. To medical historians, this superficially shocking admission will be no surprise. In peacetime, military medical systems preparation for combat directly competes for resources with delivery of peacetime medical care. Without the push from the emergency of war, there never seems to be time for full training or planning.

This problem, at least in Europe, extended even into the combat divisions. Although divisions have an excellent organic mental health team consisting of a psychiatrist, social worker, psychologist, and at least five behavior science specialists, in Europe division mental health professionals are usually under pressure to provide local community mental health service rather than train or plan for war. Furthermore, in many cases the most junior clinicians are assigned to divisions and are often less effective than they would be with more rank and more military experience.

A further detractor from psychiatric combat readiness, true both historically and in the Gulf War, is that medical teams for war tend to be created or changed at the moment of crisis. In the two European divisions which deployed to the Gulf, only three of the six officers who deployed were in place before the war, and several enlisted behavioral science specialists were changed at the last moment.

When the war began, the 7th MEDCOM psychiatric consultant gave highest priority to design of a psychiatric annex to the wartime operational plan (OPLAN) and to support of formation of division mental health teams. Because of pressure from the war, an annex was rapidly accepted which would have required a vastly more complex and time-consuming staffing process had it been submitted in peacetime. Divisions at the onset of the war had many mental health personnel shortages. Coordinated work among the 7th MEDCOM psychiatric, social work, and psychology consultants helped complete the division teams using cross-leveling of mental health officers and enlisted personnel from other areas in Europe.

The psychiatric consultant, the social work consultant, and the commander of the U.S. Army Medical Research Unit Europe (USAMRUE) visited mental health teams of deploying divisions to help their personnel review basic combat stress consultation and treatment plans. In addition, the commander of USAMRUE, thanks to extensive networking with line commanders in the course of earlier behavioral science research, gave presentations of basic combat mental health principles to nondivisional units about to deploy.

During the war, only two nondivision psychiatrists deployed from Europe, but they were selected early. The chief of psychiatry at one of the hospitals became the psychiatrist in an evacuation hospital. The chief of psychiatry at another hospital went to an unofficial position, requested by the VII Corps surgeon, as VII Corps psychiatric consultant. The assignment of a psychiatrist to an unrecognized position met with great resistance from the personnel system, but it took place because it had support of the corps commander. Deployment was a surprise for both of these psychiatrists, and they had to manage the same ambivalent pride and shock which faced so many deploying health care providers in Europe. Neither imagined that, in a contingency operation, they would leave their hospitals in Europe for a combat zone on another continent.

The 7th MEDCOM psychiatric consultant participated in other personnel planning, including providing recommendation for the deployment of reserve psychiatrists and other mental health professionals throughout hospitals in Europe. Eventually, a substantial number of reserve psychiatrists, social workers, psychologists, behavioral science specialists, psychiatric technicians, and psychiatric nurses arrived in Europe from the United States and were distributed widely, with emphasis on support to three hospitals expecting to receive psychiatric casualties. In addition, in coordination with consultants from other mental health professions, informal planning took place to create a "hip pocket" OM team (a corps asset, consisting of 50 plus mental health professionals). Early in the war, it was not clear what mental health resources would go from CONUS to the Gulf, so it was considered possible that, on short notice, Europe would be told to compose a corps level mental health team. The team was never called.

During the early stages of the Gulf War, the psychiatric consultant had several phone conversations with the senior Army physician and the psychiatric consultant in Saudi Arabia, as well as the psychiatric consultant at the Office of the Surgeon General in Washington. These calls were helpful, but were not as extensive as desirable because of difficulties in establishing secure phone contact.

Before the ground war phase began, all mental health teams at the U.S. Army–Europe (USAREUR) hospitals trained and prepared to receive casualties. A fortunate coincidence gave them a major training aid: after years of work, the senior psychiatrist at the Academy of Health Science distributed a draft of the new combat stress control field manual FM 8-51, *Combat Stress Control in a Theater of Operations*, a monumental compendium of combat psychiatric knowledge. Although it had no official status, it was distributed to all the USAREUR hospitals and divisions. In addition, the 7th MEDCOM psychiatric consultant made multiple consultative visits to hospitals, especially those expected to receive psychiatric casualties from the Gulf.

A Department of the Army–level decision was made early in the Gulf War to continue delivery of peacetime medical care at full levels even in the face of preparation to receive massive numbers of wartime casualties. Requests for deployment of medical reservists to Europe were influenced by a desire to maintain care in USAREUR at peacetime levels while simultaneously planning for wartime patient scenarios. During the air war phase, there were in fact numerous psychiatric evacuations from the Gulf region, but it was the impression of all concerned that psychiatric evacuations were not at a rate substantially higher than would have been the case had the same troops been in garrison in the United States. An unusual benefit from the location of the war in a Moslem country where alcohol was generally unavailable was that there were almost no patients evacuated from the Gulf for consequences of alcohol abuse. The only exceptions were several unexplained seizure patients early in the war.

Even under ideal circumstances, not all psychiatric priorities can be met. After visits with psychiatrists at various 7th MEDCOM hospitals and after participation in a great number of planning activities at the 7th MEDCOM Headquarters, the psychiatric consultant sent an informal memorandum to chiefs of psychiatry at 7th MEDCOM hospitals. It suggested, but did not direct, treatment priorities. It constituted a focused one page view of all psychiatric responsibilities relevant to the war. It is reproduced here (with comments that represent subsequent observations and impressions).

USAREUR Areas of Psychiatric Responsibility during the Gulf War

USAREUR psychiatrists had seven areas of primary responsibility.

1. Treatment of psychiatric casualties. In practice, hospital commanders and staff did not put this priority as number one and were never forced to do so because there were minimal combat stress casualties. While many patients were evacuated from the Gulf, few were suffering mental problems as a consequence of combat. Most had problems similar to those of psychiatric patients under stress in peacetime, the usual mix of minor and major psychiatric diagnoses.

2. Planning for mass casualties. With the onset of the Gulf War, the USAREUR Commander in Chief directed that a new USAREUR OPLAN 4345-91, Mass Casualty/Fatality Operations be completed in record time. During the war, all of Europe was alert to the possibility of terrorist events. The OPLAN established theater-wide authority and responsibility for prompt, effective response to any disaster in Europe. It did not address, however, a new kind of mass casualty event. The new event would be the loss in war of many soldiers from a single combat unit having family members living in a single community. Were that the case, the very people who ran the unit and community family support system could themselves be included among traumatized persons, those who had lost their spouses to war. Because of other priorities, psychiatrists in USAREUR hospitals probably did not give adequate attention to planning for local disasters.

3. Mental health care to our normal peacetime population. It was mandated by the Secretary of Defense that the level of medical care traditional in Europe during peacetime not be significantly decremented during the war. In fact, with creative plans in their outlying clinics, the three hospitals destined to receive most casualties from the Gulf maintained good capacity to treat outpatients and were able to use other hospitals for inpatient services. Because patients receiving mental health care are less able to receive good care at distant locations, informal license was given to psychiatrists to continue local care at a level not true for some other specialties. Continuity of psychiatric care at the hospitals was in fact no burden because the presence of reservists, in many cases, made available psychiatric resources better than in peacetime.

4. Contributing to the family support program. Senior leaders recognized very early in the war that soldier morale hinged not only on the usual training, leadership, and small unit cohesion, but equally on the soldier's faith that his or her family would not suffer during the deployment. USAREUR went to great lengths at all levels and in all communities to design proactive family support systems of the highest quality. While the medical system did not have primary responsibility for the family support program, it gave full support to these efforts. In practice, psychiatrists were not as involved as social workers in the family support system, but were available for a variety of tasks when asked. Among psychiatrists, child psychiatrists contributed the most to the family support system and in support of local school programs designed to make the school part of the larger community support system.

5. Consultation/liaison (C/L) to medical/surgical casualties. This priority should be obvious to psychiatrists, but it was one which caught us by surprise to a degree. In practice, C/L services did take place, but were not as widespread as ideal. There were two types of patients which benefited from consultation. The first were soldiers with medical conditions which would ordinarily not cause hospitalization and evacuation, but who were sent to Europe from the Gulf because of a policy which led to the evacuation of any soldier not expected to be able to fully perform full duty in a week or less time. Psychiatrists in Europe believed that some non psychiatric patients had in fact "evacuation syndromes," genuine but minor medical conditions which enabled them to leave the combat zone prematurely. Low back pain was probably the most common of these conditions. The second types of patient, those with major medical or surgical problems, were also common and needed the same attention they would get after major illness or trauma in peacetime. Psychiatrists were alert to a feeling in many soldiers that evacuation constituted "letting down one's buddies." Other evacuated patients were glad to be out of the combat zone. In light of the spectacular allied victories in the Gulf War, we would anticipate any soldiers evacuated out of theater for minor illness would be at risk of self esteem problems in the future.

6. Support to health care providers under extreme stress. Military psychiatrists know how much stress their medical peers can fall under during times of mass casualty, particularly when stress is for a sustained period. Mental health professionals can support their medical peers by enforcing sleep discipline, encouraging cathartic discussions in supportive groups, and engaging in other activities that provide psychosocial support. The fact this priority is so low on this list only reflects that higher priorities either involve direct patient care or greater demand by outside authority. It is well known that medical personnel usually don't request stress management, but respond well to it when it is received. Unfortunately, psychiatrists believed that, had the war turned against us and we received massive numbers of psychiatric casualties, they would have had little time to implement this priority.

7. Attention to returning soldiers and their families after the war. Most reunions of soldiers and their families went well in Europe. There were minimal cases of subsequent PTSD, as would be expected in a short, successful war with minimal casualties, home front support, and great soldier pride. Two groups at risk were those who were or knew victims of friendly fire, and those who witnessed especially horrible examples of the consequences to the enemy of allied firepower. Of interest in Europe was the observation from some psychiatrists that, for many soldiers who returned from the Gulf War to Europe, stress they and their families experienced from deployment was no more than stress they experienced from uncertainties of force reductions started before the war and continued after it.

SOME AFTERTHOUGHTS

There is one more priority which was overlooked on this list: research. The 7th MEDCOM psychiatric consultant had a research psychologist as an assistant, who designed a research project focused on obtaining extensive demographic and clinical data on all psychiatric patients sent to Europe from the Gulf. Unfortunately, there was very little institutional support for this effort, and relevant clinical data were never collected.

A medical system which is stretched to provide clinical care (true of all medical systems in war) almost always gives research minimal, or even a negative, priority (i.e., actively discourages it). Rarely within a clinical medical system is there a request from higher authority for research, particularly psychiatric research. During the Gulf War, even in the face of substantial additional resources from reservists and official directives written by the psychiatric consultant and signed by the 7th MEDCOM chief of staff, departments of psychiatry resisted dedicating resources to research. Research should be given a place and credibility in OPLANs, and even it is if low on priority lists, it should always be included.

SUMMARY

Some of the points made in this chapter are necessarily sketchy and incomplete, but they accurately indicate issues which the psychiatric consultant considered important during the war. They also give an overview which any future psychiatric planner for war needs to compare with his or her own viewpoints. There are only two regrets, one legitimate and one illegitimate but psychologically valid. The first regret is that peacetime medical care realities, historical and probably future, always seem to preclude psychiatric combat readiness for a "come as you are" war. Most of the psychiatric planning described here was done after the start of the Gulf War.

The second regret is the ambivalence felt by so many medical soldiers who treated so few casualties after so much preparation. No health care provider would consciously wish for more casualties, but all health care providers take pride in successfully managing medical crises. Psychiatrists and their mental health colleagues in Europe cannot be certain how well the execution of their plans would have worked in a worst case war. They believe it would have been outstanding, but they will always wonder.

4

Psych Force 90

L. Steven Holsenbeck

INTRODUCTION

This chapter is about leadership of a field medical unit, the 528th Medical Detachment, whose mission was the prevention and treatment of battle fatigue among American combat forces during the Persian Gulf War. Psych Force 90 was the banner chosen by the members of this unit.

This chapter highlights the experiences of a field medical detachment, called an OM team (OM does not really stand for anything; it is just a standard Army unit identifier). OM teams have the mission of combat stress casualty prevention and treatment, commonly referred to as combat stress control (CSC). The organization and staffing of the standard OM team includes 48 soldiers (15 mental health officers and 33 enlisted specialists). The team is organized with a headquarters section, (three mental health officers and four enlisted specialists), one treatment team, and three consultation teams. The OM team is a corps-level unit, attached to a medical brigade or medical group headquarters, with responsibility for providing direct CSC services to non-divisional units within the corps as well as CSC back-up support to division CSC teams.

The CSC assets in a theater of operations earn their keep by preventing unnecessary personnel losses due to stress. This goal is accomplished by providing consultation and education to leaders and soldiers on stress management and first-aid for stress induced dysfunction. It is further served by early assessment and forward treatment of stress casualties, resulting in rapid return to duty. Within weeks of the deployment of the first combat troops to Saudi Arabia during the initial phase of the Gulf War, stress casualties were being returned to Army hospitals in Europe and to the United States for treatment. Early deployment of a Mobile Area Surgical Hospital (MASH) and a Combat Support Hospital (CSH) to Saudi Arabia did little to stem the steady flow of psychiatric evacuations, as neither hospital had the capability to evaluate or treat stress casualties. This loss of personnel, with minor psychiatric problems stemming from the adjustment difficulties, led to the activation and eventual deployment of the 528th Medical Detachment (OM).

PREDEPLOYMENT OPERATIONS

The 528th's activation marked the first time the U.S. Army has fielded a unit of this kind for a combat deployment. Officer personnel were assigned from the Professional Filler System (PROFIS), and enlisted personnel were drawn from the U.S. Army's Health Services Command. The 52 personnel assigned represented 23 different Army medical facilities. Except for a few volunteers, these selections were essentially random.

The commander originally designated under the PROFIS system did not arrive. A second unit commander (the author of this chapter) was designated on September 17, 1990 but did not actually arrive until September 19, 10 days after most other unit members had reported to Fort Benning. To add to the confusion, the names of other potential commanders had been informally announced to the waiting unit at Fort Benning. Throughout the life of the unit, members repeatedly referred to this two week period with irritation. It set the stage for suspicions about the reliability of support from "higher up." It also created a difficult situation for the command and staff of those host units with responsibility for bringing the 528th to deployment readiness status.

The expected date of departure for Saudi Arabia was only a week in the offing when I arrived to assume command of the 528th. Readiness for deployment is determined primarily on the basis of availability of equipment and personnel. With my arrival, the unit automatically achieved the status of combat ready and was cleared for departure. This rapid upgrade undermined unit confidence in "higher ups" while escalating the anxiety of unit members.

I assessed the situation as a genuine crisis. In the midst of the fantasies and fears driving those within and without the unit, it was paramount to establish quickly flesh and blood commander did exist. A Commander's Call was held a few hours after my arrival, in which I shared with the entire unit my relevant experience, acknowledged the gaps in my current knowledge of the detachment's status and immediate future, and conveyed my confidence that I was capable of leading the unit, with their cooperation and assistance.

Immediately following this Commander's Call, I held a separate Officer's Call, at which my officers were asked for their assessment of the most pressing problems and for their ideas regarding the best assignment of personnel on hand within the detachment. I also met the commanders and key staff of the units responsible for the detachment's preparation in order to get a status briefing and to assert a command presence with them. The two immediate higher headquarters

(Headquarters, Forces Command, and Headquarters, Health Services Command) involved in activation and deployment of the detachment were also contacted.

I then turned my attention to an assessment of the strengths and weaknesses of each unit member in an effort to balance these throughout the organization and to identify problems requiring immediate attention.   The officers and the first sergeant had interviewed each soldier individually and observed them for a few days. Their observations had been taken into account for assignment of personnel to teams within the detachment.   It was critical to settle the issue of team membership immediately so that cohesion-building processes could begin.

Finally, as the commander, I decided to assign the senior Medical Service Corps officer, a social worker, as the unit's executive officer. He was the only lieutenant colonel in the detachment and was well known and respected by several other unit officers. However, his assumption of administrative tasks reduced the unit's overall clinical capability. I also decided that the clinical psychologist, who would normally be assigned to the headquarters, would be most useful for his diagnostic and acute treatment skills in one of the consultation teams. Rare cases requiring psychological testing could be referred to him there.

It was apparent that the detachment was still not combat ready. Therefore, the final issue requiring my immediate attention was to assert this fact to those responsible for the decision to deploy the unit to Saudi Arabia. This opinion was very unpopular with the commanders of the supporting units, not to mention higher headquarters. It may have been their assumption that the decision to delay the detachment's deployment had less to do with the unit's state of readiness than with the fear that the commander was either incompetent or a fool. In any case, we gained an additional four weeks of training and preparation time.

Having won reprieve from immediate deployment, the focus shifted to developing the leadership of the organization, training all soldiers in critical survival and professional skills, and building cohesion and morale. Cohesion forms most readily in a group of 6 to 12 members. It is this primary group membership that supports the soldier under stress.   In view of the limited predeployment time available for this critical process, I made a conscious decision to focus cohesion building at the team rather than at the detachment level. The other consideration in doing this was the possibility that teams might have to deploy independently (away from the detachment headquarters).

Next to food, information is the most precious commodity in a soldier's life. The best information available must constantly be sought out and promptly passed to the soldier. It must be through the legitimate chain of command, if that chain is to maintain credibility.   Rumor must be actively sought out and dispelled. Accurate, timely information enhances legitimate authority and supports cohesion building.

My view of the critical importance of cohesion and information management in the early development of the detachment was communicated and discussed repeatedly by the command and control organization of the unit. Command and staff briefings were held daily. Team meetings were held immediately afterward so that information was rapidly and accurately disseminated. I also began a weekly Commander's Call for all members of the detachment. Separate officers, NCO, and junior enlisted calls were held every other week. This standard of communication, set early, was perhaps the most important key to the ultimate unit success.

Within two weeks, the day-to-day function of the unit had fallen into a routine, and a sense of membership, pride, and confidence had begun to grow. The desired positive momentum had been attained.

At this point in predeployment preparation, mandatory training provided by the base installation was drawing to a close, and the detachment's training schedule was increasingly in my hands as the commander. The major task from this point until departure (which was still unknown to us) was to focus training on the most essential survival skills and overall mission readiness.

The survival aspect was straightforward, although few individuals in the detachment had any field experience. Some had never even spent a night outdoors. The simplest elements of fieldcraft, such as tent pitching, vehicle loading, and field sanitation were completely new to most. Under the eye of the few with good field skills, the rest trained enthusiastically and repeatedly in these mundane but essential skills. The imminence of deployment was conducive to paying serious attention. The training was enjoyable and rewarding in the context of this realism. Despite this initial success, it is unconscionable that medical soldiers of considerable rank and time in service should be totally lacking in skills that most would consider the essence of soldiering. It is equally unconscionable that many medical soldiers were sent to a combat zone without the opportunity to develop these basic soldier skills.

Readiness for the detachment's professional mission was hindered by having only the vaguest notion of what that mission might be. Combat psychiatry is most certainly not just clinic psychiatry in a tent. That myth is responsible for many of military psychiatry's most serious credibility problems.

The greatest obstacle for the 528th was the lack of information regarding the medical context in which the unit would be expected to operate in Saudi Arabia. This was a direct result of the inability to communicate with the headquarters which would receive the unit upon deployment. Training was directed at the most likely scenarios and at those skills which were the least used in peacetime hospital practice. Three areas were identified: the occupational model, command consultation and education, and identification and management of combat stress casualties.

In contrast to the occupational model, peacetime psychiatry generally operates on the illness model, shared with the rest of medicine. It is symptom focused. The occupational model is work focused. An impaired ability to work is the problem, usually caused by adaptational difficulties in the worker and rarely caused by psychiatric disease. Treatment is focused on restoration of occupational function.

When the soldier is able to return to work, treatment is terminated, regardless of the continued presence of symptoms. This utilitarian model is the most effective model in a deployed army. The mental health tasks are to diagnose major psychiatric disease that would eliminate the possibility of a return to duty (psychoses, severe major depression) and to enhance adaptation to work oriented demands.

Command consultation and education are the primary techniques available for influencing combat stress. One of the most important areas of emphasis is the effort to enhance small unit leadership. Leadership is the key to cohesion and morale; therefore, it is a vehicle for sustaining soldiers against the stress of combat, thus preventing psychological breakdown. A cohesive, confident band of buddies is the most supportive and adaptive context for a soldier in combat. Leadership is largely a learned art, and sensitivity to the interpersonal underpinning of an effective combat unit is an acquired skill.

A variety of interventions can be used to sharpen a leader's sensitivity and ability to constructively influence cohesion and morale. Simple education, in the form of briefings and classes, is one tool. Such classes have the advantage of reaching a large audience. Their impact largely depends on the interest and openness of the leaders in the audience, as classes provide little opportunity for one on one interaction with participants. To be effective, a mental health officer presenting these classes must be both knowledgeable and a bit of a showman.

Informal consultation with leaders, of the "coffee pot" variety, is another technique. This type of consultation requires proximity, time, and social skills but is very effective. For these reasons, coffee-pot consultation is primarily used within one's own command.

Another major tool is classical, client focused or event focused consultation, in which a stress impaired soldier or a stressful group event (i.e., an accident or death) is used as a springboard for a fuller assessment of and intervention in the stress absorbing qualities of a unit. This technique can incorporate educational interventions, coffee-pot consultation, and a variety of group and individual interventions. The critical incident and combat debriefing techniques widely used in the Persian Gulf War are examples of this type of consultation.

These three techniques were taught and discussed in a series of didactic and practical training exercises during the final weeks before our deployment. This training continued in Saudi Arabia, and many of the 528th personnel developed outstanding consultation skills. Each technique requires somewhat different abilities, but one or another technique was within the capability of nearly every soldier in my unit. Soldiers assigned to consultation teams had the most opportunity to develop these skills, but everyone had an opportunity for cross training.

The final professional training task was the acquisition of the requisite skills for recognizing and treating combat stress casualties. Colonel James Stokes, author of a training module in use at the Army Academy of Health Sciences, was solicited to come to Fort Benning to conduct a full day's training. The instruction consisted of didactic sessions, discussion periods, and practical exercises. Because it incorporated many basic skills in daily peacetime use by soldiers like those assigned to the 528th, it was easily assimilated.

The detachment finally acquired a window for departure. While this event heightened anxiety, it also lent additional purpose to our activities. There was a unanimous request to return to the weapons range for an additional day of weapons training. It was clear that acquiring confidence with the individual weapon had significant symbolic and anxiety binding value for all unit members.

As the window for departure drew near, concerns increasingly turned to those being left behind. An opportunity was created to release everyone who wanted to visit home a last time. I also sent a personal letter to as many relatives and friends as each soldier designated, in which I conveyed my responsibility for the safety of the detachment's soldiers. This was an attempt to allay some of the anxieties shared by those who would watch and wait.

When the unit finally deployed to Saudi Arabia on October 26, 1990, there were still only 38 personnel assigned (Table 4.1). The unit was short one psychiatrist and nine enlisted psychiatric specialists; therefore, only two of three consultation teams were capable of fully independent operations. By existing doctrine, at least two such detachments were required to support the population in theater in late October, and that population in Saudi Arabia was growing by over 8,000 personnel every 24 hours. Nevertheless, our higher headquarters insisted that the 528th would deploy with no more than the standard fill. Three months later, on the eve of combat, the population in theater had quintupled. The 528th still had only 38 personnel.

Table 4.1
528th Medical Detachment (Desert Shield), 38 Personnel (14 OFF and 24 ENL)

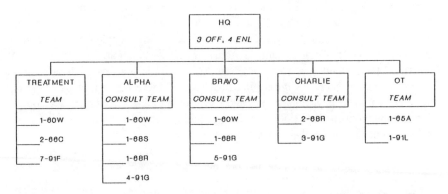

This lengthy discussion of the predeployment period underscores the old maxim, "Preparation is nine tenths of execution." The group culture which emerged at Fort Benning proved adequate for everything the detachment eventually faced. That culture was the product of the individuals involved and the situation that brought them together, and in that regard was a culture shared by many other deploying units. It was also a culture shaped by application of certain leadership principles and techniques.   It evolved as key leaders found commonalties of principle, as a shared vision of a model detachment developed out of input from above and below, and as the cauldron of anticipation and anxiety melded unit members into a single, bonded entity.

THE BUILDUP PHASE OF THE PERSIAN GULF WAR: OPERATION DESERT SHIELD

Arrival in Saudi Arabia was disorienting. The detachment had no instructions concerning expected actions upon arrival. A chance conversation over the first meal in the country provided an opportunity to meet the senior medical officer in our Corps, the Commander of the 44th Medical Brigade of the XVIII Airborne Corps. He confirmed that the 528th was the only psychiatric entity in theater except for the division mental health teams of the lst Cavalry, 101st Air Assault, and 82nd Airborne Divisions.

On October 28, 1990, general mission taskings were assigned based on the distribution of troops in theater and the capabilities of the 528th. These initial orders conveyed the first of many surprises to the detachment's leaders. As I had feared, the detachment would not be able to operate out of a single site. Such a split deployment was inherent in the design of the detachment. However, only brief, roving consultation team trips afield had been envisioned, operating out of a detachment base camp. The specter of semi-permanent banishment to the desert came as a shock to everyone in the unit.

A recon trip was immediately organized. This trip, involving the two leaders of the teams affected, swiftly restored confidence in the detachment's ability to meet the challenge. The chance to walk the land and meet the people with whom they would be living and working set team leaders at ease and recast the tasking into an adventure. The impressive sight of an entire corps encamped in the desert did much to dispel the sense of danger. On their return, both team leaders were able to generate enthusiasm for the operation. When their preparations were completed, each team received a hearty send-off from those who remained behind.

By November 3, 1990, the detachment's treatment team had 20 holding cots operational, and one consultation team had begun command consultation and outpatient triage in the Dhahran area. By November 14 the two other consultation teams were operating in the forward area of the corps, approximately 150 miles from Dhahran. Between November 3, 1990 and January 10, 1991, the detachment logged 600 unit consultations and 387 psychiatric evaluations and held 123 soldiers for treatment.

Throughout the build-up phase, the detachment's energy was directed toward two priorities: sustainment of day to day operations and further preparation for war.   Day to day operations of the three consultation teams consisted of two primary activities: command consultation and psychiatric triage. The conduct of command consultation consisted of actively seeking opportunities to advise and educate commanders and soldiers on the identification, command management, and "buddy aid" of stress induced dysfunction. Both patient referrals and critical incidents were followed up by team members with offers of consultation and combat stress training. Critical incidents consisted of a variety of circumstances which might be expected to induce stress related dysfunction, such as training accidents, or which might be manifestations of high unit stress, such as the discharge of a weapon in anger. Consultations with command were aimed at identifying correctable sources of stress—unrealistic work-sleep schedules, for instance—and advising on their management. Combat stress training (including precombat stress associated with the deployment) was directed at increasing the capability of individuals and units to adapt to stressors which were not readily correctable, such as heat stress or continuous operations. The availability and effectiveness of command consultation was quickly advertised by word of mouth, resulting in far more requests for consultation and combat stress training than the detachment could fulfill.

The second primary day-to-day activity of the consultation teams was triage of dysfunctional soldiers.   Conditions dictated that these interventions usually be limited to a single session. The purpose of triage was to identify major mental illness, which necessitated consideration of evacuation from theater, and/or life threatening behavior, which necessitated consideration of holding for treatment. Otherwise, soldiers were provided an opportunity to ventilate on the spot. The problem was refocused in terms of those elements within their power to influence here and now. Their chain of command was consulted on unit actions, both in theater and, when the problem involved family issues, at the home station.

Those soldiers who exhibited life threatening behavior, or were too disruptive to remain in their units, or were awaiting aeromedical evacuation from theater were held in cots in tents in a military atmosphere which emphasized healthy functioning through an intensive occupational therapy program and promoted adaptation through psychoeducational classes and small group therapy.   The emphasis was always on limited ventilation of emotions, restructuring of the problem into here and now resolvable issues, and acquisition of adaptational skills combined with active command consultation.

During the build up phase, the total number of soldiers who benefited directly or indirectly from unit consultations reached at least several thousand. Only 150 of the soldiers held for treatment were ultimately evacuated from the combat theater. These soldiers constituted less than 6 percent of all soldiers triaged by the detachment. For the most part, soldiers brought to the detachment for triage had already failed other attempts at problem resolution and, in many cases, had also failed interventions at other echelons of medical and/or mental health care. They represented only a small and more dysfunctional portion of the total number of soldiers who were temporarily dysfunctional within the theater during the Persian Gulf War.

In this period of relatively stable operations, each team was acquiring its own unique body of experience and its own identity, separate from the other teams and from the parent detachment. Team members were realizing the strengths and weaknesses of teammates, and complementary roles were evolving. Additionally, each team was experiencing the rewards of its own successes, with steadily increasing credibility and esteem among the commanders and units they served. A competitive spirit developed between teams as each convinced itself that it was the best in the detachment. The detachment headquarters even came to be perceived as the enemy on occasion. Howls of protest erupted when teams were asked to share equipment or supplies.

In general, each team's maturation toward independence was a healthy and essential process. As will be discussed later, each team ultimately had to function in a setting almost entirely independent of the rest of the detachment. The tensions created at the boundaries between teams, and between each team and the headquarters, however, were counterproductive. These were products not only of success but also of ongoing anxiety about war and of envy (in a sense, this was a form of sibling rivalry). Moderating these regressive forces required active attention from the commander, first sergeant, and team leaders. Verbal reminders of the integrity of the detachment as a whole kept the issue in focus. Detachment celebrations at Thanksgiving, Christmas, and New Year's, to which members of the desert teams were invited, helped maintain camaraderie. Cross training of personnel between the "desert" consultation teams and the treatment team fostered mutual appreciation of each other's particular hardships. The most nagging problem for the detachment was its inability to perform certain daily survival functions for itself. The staffing did not include personnel for vehicle maintenance or food service. The inadequacy of the command and staff element has already been mentioned. These three shortfalls in capability compounded each other in that inordinate amounts of the detachment leaders' time was absorbed in the mundane but essential task of ensuring that all members of the detachment were fed and watered and had functioning transportation.

Coordination of mess and vehicle maintenance support for the widely dispersed detachment elements required constant attention. The detachment eventually acquired some autonomy in the supply area when it was granted purchasing authority and allowed to requisition directly from the various supply points. Stabilization of relationships with supporting units throughout this period helped the messing problem, but vehicle maintenance and access to spare parts continued to be a nuisance.

In addition to day-to-day operations, the detachment was actively preparing for war. Several attempts were made to obtain the additional combat stress control resources that standard planning factors indicated were needed to conduct offensive operations. While fully supported by the corps, these resources were not forthcoming. As the commander, I was confronted with the task of somehow expanding the detachment's holding capability by a factor of 10. This necessity was not, at first, apparent to higher headquarters. While the commander of the 44th Medical Brigade (our immediate commander) appreciated the importance of combat stress control efforts, the brigade staff was largely uneducated about the mission, capability, and potential requirements for combat stress control services in various combat scenarios. Many hours of formal briefings and coffee pot consultation went into a painstaking educational process.

A case example will illustrate a number of points. In December, two newly arrived medical group headquarters elements came under control of the medical brigade. All medical units which had heretofore come directly under brigade control, as well as the additional medical units coming into theater to support the offensive, were to be reorganized under one of these two group headquarters. One, the lst Medical Group, was to manage forward medical support of the XVIII Airborne Corps offensive. The other group was assigned the rear area and was composed primarily of large evacuation hospitals. It was to set up at airheads in Saudi Arabia and function as treatment and transfer points for the more severely wounded, who were lost to battle and were being evacuated out of theater. The initial order for task organization of the brigade placed the 528th in the rear area medical group. This decision was taken in spite of the fact that U.S. doctrine for the management of combat stress casualties since World War II has been to treat them as far forward in the battle area as possible. The principles of proximity, immediacy, and expectancy were, in fact, first applied in World War I. Assigning the detachment to a location far in the corps rear, at the end of a long evacuation chain, hundreds of miles from the units to which over stressed soldiers should return, contradicted everything taught about combat stress casualty management for 70 years. Doctrine would place the OM team with the forward most medical elements of the corps, or even collocated with division medical elements. In the end, the faulty thinking in the task organization was confronted, and the detachment was moved to the lst Medical Group, where it served out the remainder of the operation.

While war plans changed every few days, two factors emerged early and clearly. The 528th was all the corps was going to have, and many casualties were expected. Reorganization for combat was critical to our success in treating the number of combat stress casualties estimated under the planning guidance provided by the corps. The detachment's holding capability was only 25 cots; that had to be expanded to 240 cots. Mission success would require reorganization of the treatment and consultation specialty teams into hybrids that could each perform consultation, triage, and treatment holding equally well. It called for cross leveling of critical nursing and occupational therapy personnel and crosstraining of all enlisted personnel. It required the acquisition of tentage, vehicles, and other equipment needed to support the additional patient load. Efforts were also launched to obtain personnel and equipment augmentation from within theater by tapping other mental health assets with less critical missions. These initiatives did not come to fruition until just weeks, in some cases days, before the ground war commenced.

During November, preparations focused on intensive nuclear, biological, and chemical (NBC) defense training, combat stress casualty management skills, further acquisition of field operating skills, environmental threat management (physiological adaptation and preventive medicine), and equipment familiarization and maintenance. As offensive plans took shape in December, the focus of preparation shifted to functional reorganization of the detachment, cross training of organic personnel, combat role definition, and development of standing operating procedures for management of large numbers of combat stress casualties. These preparations continued during the air campaign of the Persian Gulf War.

Another key function of the detachment during this build up phase was coordinating the psychiatric teams in the evacuation hospitals, as well as coordinating and supporting to the division combat stress teams in the theater. A significant part of this function was to educate uninformed mental health personnel regarding the principles of combat psychiatry and their implementation in this theater. Many lacked the knowledge and skills necessary for effective functioning in their wartime roles; this was true of active component personnel as well as reserve component personnel.

Monthly mental health meetings were sponsored by the detachment. Transportation was provided for those without means to attend. Because of the distances involved, attendees often stayed overnight with the detachment.

Support to other mental health sections often included using the influence of the detachment commander to obtain better support from that section's parent headquarters. Briefings, coffee pot consultations, repeated visits, and outright entreaties on behalf of the combat stress mission were all used to get the most out of the inadequate resources in theater.

Unfortunately, problems with professional personnel selection and preparedness were prevalent throughout the medical forces, especially in the area of medical leadership. Except for the medical brigade and group commanders, most of the other medical commanders were physicians who had been acquired from the Professional Filler System. Few of these physicians had been selected with any attention to their ability or motivation to lead others in a combat environment. A few were outstanding, most were mediocre, and others were outright failures. In many medical units, the cost in terms of morale and efficiency was high. Unfortunately, outspokenness did not correlate with leadership ability. Some of these inept leaders made life difficult for all because of the intensity with which they defended their faulty ideas about combat medical support.

On the positive side, the competence and maturity of the detachment personnel continued to improve, as did their versatility, due to cross training. Morale and cohesion remained high in spite of the rigors of daily living and the anticipation of war. As experience accumulated, the unit became increasingly effective. This effectiveness was recognized by its consumers whose praise and confidence in the "product" boosted morale and fueled efforts to achieve the highest levels of competence.

THE GROUND COMBAT PHASE OF THE GULF WAR

This phase opened with the staged repositioning of the detachment's teams to the tactical assembly areas of the XVIII Airborne Corps far to the west of our original positions and up against the border of Iraq. The hybrid combat stress treatment/consultation teams of the 528th were now under the operational control of surgical task forces hybridized from the CSHs and MASHs in the 1st Medical Group. This concept was conceived through the realization that the offensive envisioned by the corps was not supportable with the heavy, slows-moving hospitals in the inventory. Fast, light medical task forces that performed little other than triage, surgical stabilization, and further evacuation were all that was essential. With priority going to the support of the combat force, there was not food, water, or fuel for anything but the minimum essential services to save lives. The major exception was that medical element with the greatest capability of restoring temporarily ineffective soldiers to duty quickly: combat stress treatment/consultation teams.

With the entire Central Army on the move and the clear message to U.S. troops that the way home was through Iraq, requirements, as well as opportunities, for patient care and unit consultation diminished. The detachment's central focus during the 43 days of the air campaign was final preparation for the ground war.

In addition to continued unit training, preparations broadened to include three new tasks: training and integration of augmentees and filler personnel; coordination of the corps combat stress plan; and cross training of nonpsychiatric medical personnel to assist in the combat stress mission. The first of these tasks fell to the team leaders. Additional personnel finally began to arrive. Team leaders became responsible for the intensive effort required to bring 21 new members to a state of confident readiness. They had only a few days to achieve what had taken four months with the original 38 personnel. Moreover, the natural reluctance of the original team members to incorporate strangers into their tightly cohesive groups on the eve of war had to be worked through. Table 4.2 details the composition of the team during the Desert Storm (ground combat) phase of the Gulf War.

To enhance this integration, I took several measures. First, I personally went to the replacement station to pick up each newly arrived soldier to emphasize his or her importance to the detachment. If new soldiers already knew someone in the detachment, they were assigned to the same team. If new soldiers had already become buddies with another new soldier in their contingent, the two were assigned together. I personally observed training for new personnel. Problems with their acceptance were addressed aggressively. Great effort was expended on ensuring that new personnel were issued a complete set of equipment, as many had arrived without flak jackets and other protective equipment. This dedication

Table 4.2
528th Medical Detachment (Desert Storm), 38 Personnel (17 OFF and 41 ENL)

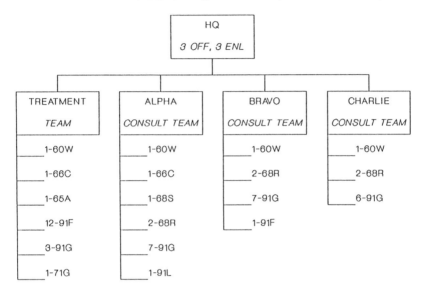

to their well being hastened their integration by instilling confidence and setting the expectation that the "old hands" would follow the commander's example.

The second task, coordination of the corps' combat stress plan, was self inflicted. As advice had not been specifically solicited by many of the players in the plan, this was a time-consuming task which required a great deal of tactful interaction at command levels. It seemed logical and necessary, though, that someone should attempt to integrate the corps' many combat stress assets. These assets included the division mental health sections of the three assigned divisions, the 528th itself, and the psychiatric sections of the five evacuation hospitals assigned to the corps. Most of the latter were newly arrived in theater and had not been included in the earlier coordination efforts. The various combat stress elements were spread over 200 miles of desert, which required several hours of on and off road travel to negotiate. Many mental health personnel at the evac hospital level had little concept of their potential role in case of combat, and they required both consultation and intensive training. Most division mental health sections were at a high level of readiness, and only coordination was required to integrate them with their supporting corps elements, primarily consisting of the teams of the 528th.

The third task, cross training of nonpsychiatric medical personnel from corps clearing companies, was part of the contingency plan to expand the combat stress treatment capability in the forward area of the corps. This contingency is critical to execution of combat stress control doctrine. Clearing companies have an additional mission of augmenting combat stress control. Once the decision was made by the 1st Medical Group Commander to assign this contingency mission to a medical battalion in the group, training was coordinated and begun with the designated clearing platoons. Clearing personnel were generally receptive and could have provided augmentation had the contingency been required.

As the 528th Commander, my emphasis during these last weeks of preparation was primarily on helping the four hybrid combat stress treatment/consultation teams achieve the proper focus to accomplish their respective missions. Each team was now essentially autonomous from the detachment headquarters and was entirely under the operational control of its respective task force commander. These were uneasy command relationships. The task force commanders were new to the "old hands" of the 528th, who had not worked with these officers previously. From the viewpoint of the task force commanders, combat stress was a poorly understood concept and being made responsible for "shrinks" was not enthusiastically received by some. Setting both sides at ease was a major task during the final weeks and was not entirely successful. The same old battles for food, water, and vehicle maintenance support had to be fought over and over.

Just days before the ground war started, a division surgeon in the corps requested that a team from the 528th be released to division control to augment his division mental health section. This is an important alternative in the consideration of combat stress control doctrine. In favor of the option is the maximization of the principle of proximity and the relative ease of return to duty while operating within the division boundaries. In the context of this division's operations plan, however, important combat stress control capabilities might have been lost. The main support battalion, where the team was proposed to operate, was envisioned as moving potentially every 12 to 24 hours. To provide any combat stress control function which the division was not already able to perform for itself, the 528th required the capability of resting soldiers for 24 to 72 hours; this would not have been possible in the division scenario offered. If the division main support battalion was not called on to move rapidly, then it would be augmented by a corps medical task force containing a combat stress team from the 528th anyway. In this case, nothing would be gained in terms of capability but much could be lost by uprooting the combat stress team on, literally, the eve of war. As commander, I decided that the 528th's teams were optimally deployed under the existing plan.

By February 24, 1991, the 528th was as ready as it could get under existing constraints. After 60 to 80 hours of continuous movement, the combat stress teams of the 528th were established with their respective task forces across central and southern Iraq in the area of operations of the XVIII Airborne Corps. By integrating into the ambulance and litter bearing teams of the task forces and circulating through the patient triage and treatment areas, combat stress team members were ideally situated to provide continuous informal consultation to medical staff and to screen incoming casualties.   Spontaneous, informal, consultative interventions were made in a variety of contexts, from a shaken aircrew which had just evacuated a load of badly injured Iraqi children, to a minimal-care ward staff split very emotionally by the need to care for wounded POWs. Screening and preventive debriefing of U.S. wounded, identification and treatment of the few cases of typical battle shock, and debriefing of English-speaking POWs were also accomplished.

The brevity of the war begs the question, "What might have been?" Obviously, the answers are pure speculation. At the point at which combat operations halted, the only communication link between the detachment headquarters and the teams was the helicopter. Unless this situation had improved, continued coordination of the combat stress plan would have been impossible. Given that the quantity of combat stress assets in the corps was inadequate to handle the combat stress casualty flow predicted by casualty estimates available just days before the war began, close coordination of combat stress control operations was critical. Had the battle generated the number of casualties predicted by the existing model, forward treatment of combat stress casualties may have disintegrated due to inadequate communications.

A combat stress casualty remains a casualty until returned to duty. Because of the brevity of combat and the small number of unwounded combat stress casualties seen, there was no opportunity to test the system's ability to return soldiers to duty. The personnel administration organization is responsible for this function, but there was little reason to believe that their plan would work. The detachment expected to have to effect return to duty without assistance from other organizations and had formulated a plan to accomplish this critical part of the combat stress mission. There was neither time nor means to put this plan into effect. The plan would have worked only if communications had improved and if the advance had slowed enough to push soldiers forward to their units safely from the detachment's locations.

Implementation of command consultation, particularly in the form of combat debriefings, was another objective which was not accomplished before hostilities ended. This mission, too, was heavily communication dependent. Due to the fluidity of the battlefield, locating units that required intervention would have been difficult and potentially hazardous early on. Had conditions stabilized and communication improved, this part of combat stress operations could have gone forward as planned in a longer war.

Under the circumstances, these activities commenced during retrograde operations with identification of critical incidents, followed by unit debriefings and command consultation.

REDEPLOYMENT

All 528th personnel had been extracted from Iraq by March 10, 1991. The period from March 10 to April 20, the date the unit deactivated at Fort Benning, Georgia, was filled with the mundane tasks of preparing personnel and equipment for shipment home. There was ample time and opportunity for detachment members to process their own experiences, both internally and with their peers. Increased access to telephones allowed for the initiation of reunions with family and friends. There were few requests for patient screening or treatment in a corps giddy with success and extremely happy to be headed home. The detachment continued to seek out pockets of trauma for early intervention and became actively involved, along with chaplains and others, in providing reunion briefings. These clinical activities were relatively limited, however, by the generally happy state of affairs and, probably, by the difficulty units had in locating us and us them in a corps rushing for home. In retrospect, this was a critical period when important preventive work could have been accomplished.

The general mood was also an obstacle. On the one hand, there was a euphoria at having ended the war so quickly and with so little loss of American lives. In this context, there was a reluctance to focus on the losses that did occur. To have been so frightened waiting for the war, one was thrown off balance when there was so little of it. Suddenly one could linger on thoughts of home, thoughts that had been warded off for months.

On the other hand, there was a letdown for many. Unfulfilled expectations, even though they were horrible expectations, left a sense of bitterness for some. Because there wasn't enough war to go around, pure chance separated those who became heroes from those who just showed up. And there was the unspeakable horror inflicted on the Iraqi people. It was difficult not to feel like a bully after having seen the rag tag bunches of ill clothed young men who constituted "the fifth largest fighting force in the world." The few who ventured to speak quietly about these sights were quickly shouted down in sudden bursts of anger.

These internal conflicts sapped the energy needed to buck the current that carried the detachment passively out of the theater. There was much more work to do and sparse resources to do it with. The will to do it just was not there. Instead, the detachment kept its place in the long line that led home. One station in this line required the submission of awards recommendations. This was the most frustrating and conflicting requirement of the whole deployment. It was painful to all to stratify the unit according to somewhat arbitrary standards of merit. This was the first wedge driven into the extraordinarily tight seam that marked the bonding of unit cohesion.

I reluctantly realized that this loosening of the unit bond was inevitable and that it should be managed carefully. Team identity had been vigorously fostered, but now it seemed wise to begin to dissipate team cohesion. The first step in this direction was a return to a more traditional living arrangement. Team members had initially shared a single tent, males and females, officer and enlisted living together. The detachment gradually shifted back to officer, NCO, and enlisted tenting, with males and females separated. This shift was welcomed by some but regretted by others. It symbolized the loss that all were anticipating when the unit dissolved on arrival back at Fort Denning.

Another deliberate action was to deemphasize team leadership and emphasize the detachment leadership. The decision was prompted by the recognition that the postwar letdown was hitting some harder than others. Particularly hard hit were some of the most enthusiastic members of the unit who, due to luck of the draw, had not had the chance to enter into operations in Iraq. Their sense of meaninglessness was profound. Immersing them in the important and detailed planning necessary to get the detachment home quickly restored their sense of purpose.

Finally, on the April 18, 1991, the detachment left Saudi Arabia and headed home. On arrival at Fort Benning, at about 0800 on April 19, the detachment found an excited crowd waiting. Then, to everyone's chagrin, the detachment was crowded into one large formation with other units arriving on the same aircraft for the welcoming ceremony. The detachment was not allowed to stand behind its own colors for one last time. The blow was compounded by the confusion which ensued when it was announced that all personnel were to board a bus to the airport immediately to catch waiting flights home. Certainly no one could turn down this chance, but most were not prepared for such a peremptory farewell to friends with whom they had shared so much.

Prior to the return, a final party at Fort Benning had been planned. This plan was discarded amid the confusion and the offer of hastily arranged flights home. This disrupted any semblance of consensus. In retrospect, this decision was probably a mistake; the soldiers would have benefited from a few days of depressurization and a chance to say unhurried good byes.

The detachment went out of existence at an impromptu formation just 24 hours after arrival back in the United States. A number of soldiers had already left for home. It was a sad and happy moment marking the end of the 528th Medical Detachment (Psychiatric).

CLINICAL REVIEW

During 171 days in theater, the 528th conducted 514 psychiatric evaluations of soldiers, of which 124 (24 percent) were held for treatment and 18 (3.5 percent) were evacuated from theater. All those not evacuated were returned to their units for duty. Command consultations totaled 811. Only a few unwounded soldiers were seen specifically for combat-related stress reactions, but more than 100 soldiers wounded or injured during the invasion of Iraq were screened in preventive interventions.

LESSONS LEARNED

The 528th made its greatest impact during the build up phase of the Persian Gulf War. Deployment of the detachment at the end of October reduced the overall psychiatric evacuation rate by at least 50 percent. The portion of psychiatric evacuations due to adjustment disorders fell from previous levels by approximately 50 percent; the portion due to personality disorders fell by more than 50 percent. Consequently, personnel evacuated for psychiatric reasons were more likely to carry a major psychiatric diagnosis.

The results argue strongly for even earlier deployment of mental health assets in future operations and also for greater attention to the readiness and deployability of the active Army's single OM team. Psychiatric evacuation was much more likely to result if a soldier sought mental health consultation from the Psychiatric Section at an Evacuation Hospital than if he or she first presented to a Division Mental Health Section or OM team.

During this build up phase, the majority of soldiers triaged were suffering adjustment difficulties. The most commonly associated factor was deployment to Southwest Asia within 90 days of assignment to a new unit. It was exceptional to see a patient for whom this was not true. This fact once again underscores the importance of group membership in preventing stress related dysfunction and points to a major cost of extensive cross leveling and the use of "filler" personnel.

Most soldiers presented for treatment within a month of arrival in theater. This points to the need for active consultation with commanders and stress management training *prior to* deployment. It also reinforces the requirement for putting mental health personnel in theater early and focusing some of their efforts on in country assembly areas. Since many of these early adjustment problems stemmed from problems at home rather than from problems in theater, continued improvement must be made in family support programs.

Other special clusters which require consideration in planning for future deployments included mothers of small children, who suffered deeply both the loss of their own bond to their child and the knowledge of the loss suffered by the child. A second cluster consisted of soldiers, largely reservists and guardsmen, who suffered chronic psychiatric disabilities which required psychotropic medications either not available in theater or contraindicated due to their potential impairment of heat tolerance. This latter group accounted for a sizable portion of those evacuated from theater. A third special group was made up of veterans of prior combat, usually senior noncommissioned officers, who experienced exacerbation of combat related trauma from prior wars. Medical personnel were over represented among soldiers triaged, but this was largely due to their proximity to sources of psychiatric care. Neurologic skills possessed by psychiatrists were found to be particularly important in identifying a number of personnel whose behavioral dysfunction was secondary to a previously undiagnosed organic condition.

The primary mental health lesson learned by the Psych Force 90 experience was the confirmation of the basic principles of combat psychiatry: proximity, immediacy, expectancy, and simplicity. Psychiatric teams were deployed close to troop concentrations (proximity), where command education and consultation could be applied and dysfunctional soldiers could be rapidly evaluated (immediacy). The expectation that psychiatric symptoms would result in early return home was removed, and psychiatric personnel exhibited confidence that most problems could be effectively managed in theater (expectancy). Application of practical crisis intervention techniques, occupationally oriented therapy, and command consultation (simplicity) resulted in a marked decline in psychiatric evacuations from theater in November and December as compared to September and October. While the impact of preventive efforts is difficult to quantify, many observers and participants believed that extensive unit training concerning combat and pre combat stresses, as well as reunion stresses, significantly reduced the incidence of stress related dysfunction. No doubt the absence of alcohol and street drugs from the environment also contributed to this result.

The design of the OM team is not flexible enough to meet the demands of AirLand Battle doctrine. Patient holding capability must be decentralized if it is to be done in the forward area of the corps, and it must be done in the forward area if return to duty is to be effected. Multiple small teams, each with consultation, triage, and holding capabilities, are required to support the corps. The 528th achieved such a configuration through reorganization and crosstraining.

The preference for ground evacuation of combat stress casualties was not supportable in the combat phase of the Persian Gulf War. The rapidity of movement of combat forces, the great distances over which battles were simultaneously fought by corps elements, and the difficulty of land navigation all mitigated against the use of ground evacuation. A compromise must be struck between the principle of proximity and the requirement for conditions under which a combat stress casualty may be held for up to 72 hours. The air ambulance has, perhaps, created a psychological proximity that must replace the old concept of geographical proximity in combat stress casualty care.

CONCLUSION

Perhaps the most important lesson to be learned by the Army Medical Department is that leadership is just as important in combat medicine as it is in combat arms. Psych Force 90 proved again that significant combat power can be conserved by applying the basic principals of combat psychiatry. It tested many of the concepts inherent in the development of new combat stress control organizations and doctrine, like the efficacy of occupational therapists in a combat stress control function. Through reorganization, crosstraining, and ingenuity, the detachment expanded its combat stress casualty treatment capability 10-fold in preparation for the ground offensive, although this was not tested. In spite of mistakes and some outright failures, Psych Force 90 deserves the careful study of leaders of combat stress control units facing deployment in future conflicts.

5

18th Airborne Corps OM Team

David C. Ruck

INTRODUCTION

This chapter builds on and complements Holsenbeck's description of Psych Force 90. It discusses the basics of mental health team building and how team roles changed with changing situations, e.g., providing area mental health coverage and consultation and unit debriefings during the cease-fire and redeployment phases of the Gulf War.

The OM team was delineated under the Army Table of Organizations and Equipment document (TOE 8-620) as one of many area and unit medical support teams. It had never been fielded before, so the whole experience was an incredible learning experience.

The construction of the headquarters section and the treatment team was relatively easy, as both required specific military occupational specialties (MOSs) which were not listed for the consultation teams. Construction of the consultation teams was more problematic, as the appropriate personnel were in short supply and those chosen were essentially unknown to each other (both officer and enlisted). Assignment to teams was based on what little knowledge was available about people (i.e., MOS, past military experience in nonmedical MOSs, merit badges [Expert Field Medical Badge, or EFMB, Airborne, Air Assault], rank and gender). A major problem confronting us was how to develop team cohesiveness (both for the OM team and its subelements).

The OM elements gained role identity as they developed and matured. The behavioral science specialists (identified by the occupational specialty code 91G) wanted to know more about their jobs than that they were supposed to do whatever they were told to do (especially because we did not really know what to tell them since most of the officers had never been assigned to field medical units). Training schedules were developed to promote flexibility; cross-training of medical enlisted skills; clinical mental health skills; brief interviews to focus on the presenting problems and avoiding detailed developmental histories; consultative skills; learning combat stress control information; combat stress management lectures and discussions; and Army skills (learned new ones or refreshed old ones)—communications, maintenance, sanitation, NBC (gas chamber), supply, administration, weapons firing, convoy and blackout driving, and vehicle painting.

The unit drew on those precious few soldiers with prior Army field skills—nonpsychiatry MOS or division mental health experience. General forging of unit and team integrity occurred with the typical dynamics of small group formation. It began with getting our "stuff"—vehicles and tents, all in lousy condition and poorly maintained. There was also unit bonding via traditional us- versus-them mentality. Initially, it was the 528th versus the custodial/parent units, then the consultation teams versus headquarters or treatment sections, and finally one consultation team versus another consultation team.

The Alpha (A) consultation team began its existence with seven members (two short of its authorization of nine) and later numbered 12 at the time of deployment into Iraq. Of the seven original members, none had prior field medical experience, although one had spent two years as a forward observer for a field artillery unit. Two mental health officers had experience dealing with nonwar crises—the aftermath of the Fort Campbell Gander Crash, and treating the survivors of the Marine Beirut Bombing at Landstuhl Army Medical Center in Germany. Of the five fillers, two had prior military experience in the military police and field artillery. The two reservists had no field medical experience as an OM team member; however, they had practical knowledge of OM team functions and vehicle maintenance and operator skills. No one had exposure to combat or even direct contact with massive trauma in civilian life.

The A team had difficulty integrating new members—trying to practice what we taught other units about decreasing potential stress by making the newcomers welcome. After denying that we needed new members (which seems ridiculous, in hindsight) with all sorts of rationalization, the team reluctantly began accepting new members in mid-January. In less than four weeks, the A team went from 7 to 12 members. The four new members from outside the 528th came in pairs. The two reserve officers came together from the United States, as did the two sergeants. They were assigned to subteams and given original team members as sponsors to help with their integration and acceptance. The team composition on leaving Fort Benning in October was a psychiatrist, a psychologist, a social worker, and four behavioral science specialists. By the time the team deployed into Iraq, a social worker, three behavioral science specialists, and one occupational therapy assistant had been added.

Combat stress control role-playing by some team members with well-thought-out scenarios and treatment decisions by the rest of the staff cemented the team's confidence. Other morale-building events were tent pitching in the dark during a light rain and finally setting up our large tent in a 50-mph (miles per hour) windstorm in Iraq after 30 hours on the road.

We attempted to build on strengths and strengthen weaknesses. Cross-training was continued and focused on consultation and education skills. While waiting for deployment into Iraq, the team drew on the medical skills of the combat support hospital staff and the medical clearing company staff to enhance basic medical skills. The best team building occurred mid February 1991, after integration of the new team members.

Once A team was collocated with a combat support hospital, it began functioning in the consultation mode for which it had trained. One mental health officer and one 91G were on call for the hospital (i.e., sick call and inpatient consults). One 91G was usually on a duty roster—guard or sanitation details. The remainder were available for area consultation/education, lectures, team maintenance, communications, weapons, and vehicle maintenance. We attempted to schedule one day off per week. The psychiatrist pulled routine sick call (0700 to 1900 hours) approximately every fifth day and night call (1900 to 0700 hours) twice a month. The basic premise for all soldiers seen was that they would return to duty unless a medically boardable condition existed, which was rare.

Soldiers (not patients) were told that life is rough here in the desert, but the way home is through Iraq. Crisis management was the focus; no in-depth evaluations or detailed developmental histories were to be performed. The team took grief from the medical staff for the apparent lack of compassion for the soldiers. Our statements that suggested that studies demonstrate that rapid return to duty prevents dysfunctional adaptation and/or possible PTSD were met with disbelief. Routine use of psychotropic drugs was avoided. Drugs which had anticholinergic side effects or which interfered with water regulation (i.e., Neuroleptics, Lithium) were particularly avoided. Soldiers were returned to duty without weapons, if necessary. The use of unit watch for suicidal soldiers was utilized when we could establish contact with the unit, but we often worked with no direct unit contact. Only occasionally was unit contact available with soldiers' units; frequently soldiers were not brought in by members of their unit, or they were brought in from the Battalion Aid Station. They usually did not know the unit field phone number, chain of command, or unit location (turn right at the third abandoned vehicle, then second left, go 1 mile, turn at hill, if you see the Bedouin tent you've gone too far). Finding units was difficult. There were few signs, terrain features were often indistinguishable, and perimeter guards frequently did not know who was on their compound let alone the one over the horizon. Units also moved suddenly without notice.

When soldiers were seen in consultation, their presenting complaints were evaluated in an attempt to determine if the problem had its onset in the desert or if it was an exacerbation of conditions which predated the deployment to Southwest Asia. Prior coping skills were evaluated whenever possible.

From mid November 1990 through early March 1991, there were 108 soldier contacts, and one civilian contractor was seen (18 combat, 28 combat support, 62 combat service support soldiers). They included 4 National Guard, 1 Army Reserve, and 103 active duty soldiers. There were 40 females and 69 males. Of these, 14 (12.8 percent) had been in the unit less than one month before deployment, and 7 (6.4 percent) had been in the unit one to three months before deployment. One combat stress casualty was assigned to his unit from Advanced Individual Training (AIT) one month prior to the start of the ground war. None of the 21 newly assigned soldiers were evacuated from the theater for psychiatric reasons.

Record keeping was fairly minimal, with a contact sheet filled out on each soldier seen. In preparation for our potential combat mission of treating combat stress casualties, diagnoses were primarily combat stress reaction—mild, moderate, hefty, or heavy. Mild and moderate diagnoses were returned to duty the same day, while hefty and heavy diagnoses were admitted to a minimal-care ward for brief observation, rest, replenishment, and treatment. The range of diagnoses covered a wide spectrum, including marital problems, somatization disorders, conversion disorders, malingering, eating disorders, sleepwalking, agoraphobia, cyclothymia, poor anger control, spontaneous miscarriage, enuresis, and cross-dressing. One evaluation was done for conscientious objector status and another for an applicant for Drill Sergeant School. In general, many of the soldiers had preexisting problems and poor coping skills, which were exacerbated (but not caused) by their deployment. The soldiers seen closely resembled the population seen in garrison division mental health or community mental health services.

Eleven soldiers were admitted for further evaluation, for a total of 52 bed days. Seven were returned to duty. Four military and the only civilian were airevacuated out of the combat theater for more definitive care, one with schizophreniform disorder (disorganized types, with a 9 to 12 month prodromal period) and four with affective disorders. One soldier was deployed on Prozac. Prior to deployment, he had been processed for a medical/physical evaluation board for depression. He deployed with his unit in part because his symptoms had improved and he was within a year of being eligible for retirement. A second soldier presented with a two to three month history of tearfulness, deteriorating work performance, preoccupation with guilt of an almost delusional nature, anorexia (with a 30 to 40 pound weight loss) and social withdrawal. (He has a strong family history of bipolar disorder [father with multiple admissions and on Lithium] and substance abuse.) The one civilian seen had been deployed with a preexisting dysthymic condition, which deteriorated after the onset of the air war, with tearfulness, decreased sleep, weight loss, tremulousness, and inability to function at work.

A fifth case will be discussed in greater detail, as it illustrates several important points about combat stress casualties—sleep deprivation, preexisting conditions, and command consultation.

CASE STUDY

The psychiatrist was called to the emergency room of the combat support hospital by the division surgeon, at 0300 hours on the day after the air war started, to evaluate A. B. (not his real initials), a senior officer in the combat arms. The patient was in his middle forties and had been brought in, against his will, for the evaluation. He had been noted to have erratic and unpredictable behavior for several weeks, which had worsened over the previous two days. He complained of decreased sleep, difficulty concentrating, occasional crying spells, and decreased appetite. He felt he did not need to come in and felt that his career was ruined. He was aware that he had been relieved of command and was angry, in a tired manner. He had fairly good reality testing. He had a very competitive nature and was several years older than his contemporaries.

He was treated according to the basic principles, with rest, reassurance, and reconstitution. He looked remarkably better after 10 hours of sleep and was asking to return to duty. He would normally have been returned to duty without other information. However, there was considerable command pressure to airevacuate him out of the area as an embarrassment to command, with corresponding reluctance on my part to airevacuate him because that was contrary to doctrine for combat stress casualty treatment.

However, further consultation with the division surgeon revealed more detailed information. The patient had had unpredictable behavior for several weeks, and he had felt unable to delegate authority. He was up all hours of the night and had told his staff to wake him up for anything (especially after a chewing out by a senior officer). He was irritable and ripped into staff members mercilessly without apparent provocation. There were frequent tearful episodes and episodes of being withdrawn or unavailable for several days in a row.

His superiors and subordinates revealed a loss of faith and trust in his abilities. He had a pervasive sense of shame and guilt associated with his loss of command. He also had poor appetite and difficulty concentrating. Based on this additional information, the decision was made to airevacuate him for treatment of his depression. Command consultation with the division surgeon stressed that this situation had been potentially preventable if proper sleep discipline had been practiced or if he had been brought to medical attention earlier.

HOW CONSULTATION WAS DONE

Two basic rules were followed: Be flexible and drink plenty of water. There was a gradual evolution of our role from the Fort Benning idea of operating from the home base of the 528th, with brief forays out and back (maybe overnight to work with corps-level units). The A team planned on supporting the nondivisional corps assets without inherent mental health assets and to function as backup for division mental health sections as needed. The initial Saudi Arabian utilization of the consultation teams was on a "corps slice" basis, with A team behind the 24th Infantry Division. The plan was to work closely with the 24th Division Mental Health sections as their continued function would allow us to cover a larger area. There also was a need to develop working relationships with the nondivisional units in the XVIII Airborne Corps Support Command (COSCOM) area. However, we did not know who they were or where they were located.

What was to be the mission of the team, to provide primary mental health coverage to the region or consultation with command? Mental health evaluations of soldiers had the potential to provide access to leadership, but most soldiers came without anyone else in their unit let alone from their chain of command. When command was accessible, feedback was given regarding the specific soldier. Inquiries were made into the overall coping of the unit and stressors particular to the unit, and offers were made for combat stress control (CSC) talks.

There was reluctance (in part from fear of the unknown) by some A team members to give the combat stress control talks. It required an essential frame shift and mind set change to go from traditional office-based mental health practice to developing an effective outreach consultation program in which team members would venture out to the units to give talks. We all had plenty of experience in having an office and waiting for people to come to us with their problems, but we had little experience going out to units and telling them they needed our services. After the initial classes led by the social worker were well received by the units, it became much easier to approach other units—both because of word-of-mouth recommendations and discovering that it was fun to give the talks.

It was surprisingly easy to get an audience for a combat stress control talk, especially as the January 1991 deadline for Iraq's withdrawal from Kuwait drew near. Combat stress control talks were certainly not a high priority for most units before August 2, 1990 or before deployment. In some ways, combat stress control was analogous to nuclear, biological, and chemical warfare talks—a necessary evil but not something one initially gave much attention. (The Medical Management of Chemical Casualty course, which was given in Dharhan at the King Fahd Military Medical Complex in November 1990, was well attended and had a waiting list, and copious notes were taken by all. The course director commented that they never had such excellent attendance during their preAugust 1990 courses.)

Our social worker was familiar with going out and knocking on doors and set up most of the unit consults. Many of these were serendipitous and developed during supply runs or maintenance trips, when the social worker got lost and talked, to whomever he found. The phone system was unpredictable, and the directions to most places were complicated at best. Several consults were set up during curbside mess hall conversations.

The three consultation teams (A, B, and C) had different experiences based on their locations and their personnel. An initial difficulty faced by all sections of the 528th was establishing working relationships with the supporting units—primarily combat support hospitals, but also mobile surgical hospitals and medical clearing companies or platoons. The OM team and subsections were not designed to function independently. There was an inadequate number of vehicles to transport all personnel and equipment; insufficient tents, cots, generators, light sets, heaters, and sundry items to perform combat stress casualty treatment and recovery at multiple sites; and no inherent maintenance, sanitation, mess hall, armorer staff, or equipment. When the teams appeared at a new location, they were often initially looked upon as an imposition, another "strap-hanger" unit with little to offer and many logistical support needs.

The A team developed a close working relationship with the combat support hospital with which it was collocated. We arrived on the first day the hospital opened for business, started receiving patients, and had its first surgical case. Going through many of their early growing pains and providing area mental health coverage helped greatly with our acceptance by them. A few preexisting acquaintances and working relationships helped ease the transition. We paid our "rent" by being integrated into the enlisted duty roster and the physicians-on-call roster for sick call and night-time emergency room coverage.

As mentioned earlier, it was difficult to move away from the medical model of providing direct patient care. But establishing our professional credibility and competence eased our acceptance by the command hospital staff. While there was resistance to receiving any combat stress control talks to be given to the combat support hospital personnel, integration of A team personnel into the frequent mass casualty exercises was more easily accepted. Appropriate combat stress were gradually introduced, and the 528th personnel were used for mental health triage, which consisted of circulating mental health teams to assess potential stress problems. Minimal-care wards were utilized for treatment of stress reactions, and cross-training of the medical staff occurred. Close affiliations were established with unit chaplains. Classes on stress were often cotaught by chaplains and A team staff.

While trying to develop a coherent plan for providing consultation to the COSCOM units in our area, we looked at which units would be at risk for developing high levels of combat stress. A generic list of types of units was compiled—medical units, graves registration (body handlers), chaplains, combat engineers, chemical companies, maintenance and transportation units, and brigade-size or larger units with no inherent mental health assets. These units were spread over a wide area. A team members performed more than 200 unit consults and traveled more than 5000 miles in less than three months.

The initial focus was on medical units; they were fairly easy to locate, they did not move often; and they had a combat stress control mission as part of their many other medical taskings. Consultation was initiated with the commander of the medical battalion, which had four medical clearing companies and one ground ambulance company. The battalion commander was aware (due to a past staff assignment at the Academy of Health Sciences) that the minimal-care beds of the clearing companies were tasked to provide care for combat stress casualties, but many of the company commanders and platoon leaders were unaware of, and less than excited about, this unexpected tasking. When informed by us, at a battalion staff meeting, of the predictions that anywhere from 10 to 50 percent of all casualties could be combat stress casualties, our entry into their companies was greatly facilitated. Over a several-week period, combat stress control classes were given to each platoon in the battalion (either by A team or B team), focusing on medical and nonmedical treatment in addition to the more general information, identification, and prevention of combat stress casualties.

As the medical assets of the XVIII Airborne Corps were aligned into medical task forces, several platoons of the clearing companies appeared to be likely elements to be collocated with the A team in support of the ground war. More effort was focused on those platoons, and close affiliations developed. Training films about combat stress were viewed and discussed. Vignettes of combat stress casualties were presented and evaluated via informal case discussions. In return, the platoons taught us basic life support skills so we could help them care for the minimally wounded or disease and nonbattle-injury cases also potentially occupying the minimal-care beds.

Several trips were made up to the 3rd Armored Cavalry Regiment (3d ACR), which had no mental health assets—not even a behavioral science specialist. Several classes were given by staff of A and B teams to personnel of the medical troop. A pediatrician and a physician's assistant were identified as the personnel who would monitor and manage the combat stress casualties for the regiment. Because of concerns about the applicability of combat stress casualty treatment doctrine to the rapidly moving medical assets of the 3d ACR, participation in a medical training exercise was arranged. Four members of A team accompanied a medical squad on a three-day field exercise. It rapidly became apparent due to the probable frequent moves (three to four per day) of the squad in support of a rapidly moving battle that ground evacuation of combat stress casualties would be unlikely. Treatment would occur in the medical troop rear area, and then only if it was likely to remain in a fixed location for a minimum of 72 hours to provide for rest and reconstitution. Efforts were then focused on prevention and identification of combat stress casualties.

Continued liaison with other mental health assets in XVIII Airborne Corps was essential Monthly meetings were scheduled at Headquarters of the 328th and coordinated by the commander to disseminate information and discuss the status of various units. Lengths of stay for various levels of care were discussed, and ideal flow of combat stress casualties was outlined. A biweekly meeting was established for the mental health assets (A team, B team, 24th Infantry Division (ID) Division Mental Health, and 1st Cavalry Division Mental Health) in the western sector of the corps. These meetings were established to maintain contact and enhance morale as well as to develop effective working relationships for A team as a potential replacement or augmentation for 24th Division Mental Health Section were it to suffer heavy casualties. It was essential that our teams be familiar with each other. The division mental health sections also needed to know where their back-up corps assets were, in case they had to evacuate combat stress casualties, as we were responsible for their overflow in addition to corps-level units in our area. The meetings were quite effective in developing camaraderie and establishing a forum for discussing the various handicaps the separate sections were operating under. It was important to ensure that all units were operating with similar treatment and evacuation plans.

After several months in Saudi Arabia, it rapidly became evident that the original configuration of the OM team into purely consultation or treatment teams would not be effective in handling even a modest 10 percent combat stress casualties/wounded-in-action ratio. The consultation teams needed to plan for a more active treatment role during combat. Another frame shift was needed to focus more on the treatment and return to duty of combat stress casualties. It was at this time that increased cross-training occurred between the outpatient and the inpatient enlisted specialists. Plans were also begun to augment the team's personnel with late-arriving replacement and filler personnel from active duty and the reserves as well as the occupational therapy assistant from the treatment section. This shift in focus was facilitated by the combat support hospital shutting down for three weeks to receive new equipment. With essentially no direct patient care responsibilities, time and energy were available to develop and formulate more detailed treatment plans.

Efforts began more energetically to convince the combat support hospital commander and later the medical task force commander of the need to provide food and shelter for combat stress casualties. Tent and cot spaces were already at a premium for the expected influx of wounded soldiers. We not only lacked tents, cots, generators, light sets, etc., but we also had no vehicles to transport casualties if we were to acquire them. In addition, the idea of expending scarce resources on what many perceived as not real casualties flew in the face of nonwartime training.   Typically, medical personnel in peacetime expended extensive effort on training to care for victims of massive trauma, who had little chance of surviving to fight again.   By stressing that combat stress casualties, if treated quickly and effectively using the principles of proximity, immediacy, expectancy, and simplicity, would indeed be in keeping with the Army medical department motto, "Conserve the fighting strength," we were able to sway the opinion more in the favor of allocating resources to treat combat stress casualties.

Life support was still problematic but less so than before.   The reality remained that if there was not enough room to provide shelter for all casualties, Combat stress casualties would have shelter before the more severely wounded soldiers.

Other administrative problems developed.   The patient administrative division and personnel officers (known as S-1/personnel staffs) were not set up effectively to return soldiers to duty (it was hard enough to return a disease nonbattle injury [DNBI] soldier to duty during the prehostility phase).   The hospital's mission was essentially to stabilize soldiers to the point at which they would be able to make it back to the next echelon of care, where they would either receive more definitive care or further stabilization.   Stays at the MASH/CSH were measured in hours rather than days; soldiers were not expected to remain overnight.   The combat stress casualty mission required the ability to provide rest and reconstitution for 72 hours or more before evacuation (doctrinally by ground).   Neither patient administration division nor the S-1 had the transportation assets to return soldiers to duty even if they or the soldiers knew where their units were located.

To accomplish its mission of providing for up to 80 combat stress casualties, A team needed to reorganize.   After many iterations and the addition of new personnel to bring the staff to 12 (four officers, eight enlisted) a treatment plan was developed.   There would be three 3-man treatment sections (one mental health officer, social worker, or psychologist and two 91Gs) and a backup/floating team of a psychiatrist, NonCommissioned Officer in Charge [NCOIC], and one enlisted administrative specialist.   Each section would be on primary call for 24 hours or until their census reached 20, whichever occurred first.   The officer would be responsible for screening and triaging of all potential combat stress casualties.   If it was determined that the soldier needed further evaluation, the physician would also perform a physical examination if it had not already been completed.   The enlisted specialists (91Gs) were to be responsible for providing access to food, shelter, orientation, and brief history taking as appropriate.   Sleep was one of the primary forms of treatment during the first day but a group debriefing was also scheduled.   One 91G in each section was responsible for effecting the return to duty of those soldiers who had recovered (approximately 30 to 50 percent per day).   The other 91G would monitor the soldiers, maintain discipline, and create a general expectation of return to duty and perpetuation of soldierly duties (hygiene, fire safety, uniforms cleaned, weapons cleaning, etc.). To help reinforce the military command system, the senior and/or highest-functioning soldier who was not yet ready to return to duty was to be placed in charge of the soldiers in the section, with the 91G functioning more as an advisor. Those not returning to duty would have work therapy assignments in groups supervised and monitored by the occupational therapy assistant (91L). The second and successive days of treatment would be structured with group debriefing, work therapy, and soldierly duties. If little or no improvement had occurred by the third day, consideration for ground evacuation to an evacuation hospital with a reconstitution program would be considered.

The backup team would be floating as appropriate. The psychiatrist would be working near the ER/triage area as well as circulating through the hospital, observing cases and evaluating stress levels of the staff. Medical-surgical consultations would be handled by the psychiatrist or the NCOIC, who would also provide liaison with patient administration and personnel sections of the hospital. The 91L was responsible for providing work therapy sites and supervising soldiers working at those sites. He would also be in charge of the return-to-duty mission of the team—locating supply points, water distribution sites, etc., where vehicles were likely to return to the rear areas of the soldiers' parent units.

In theory, that was how A team planned to function. Reality was quite different. We departed for Iraq at 0200 hours, February 25, 1990, and convoyed until about 1000 hours, on February 26, arriving at our first site in the middle of a severe windstorm. The forward surgical team, orthopedic section, two minimal-care tents (one of which was designated for combat stress casualties), and all large tents were set up over the course of several hours under trying and depressing circumstances. Setting up the large tent by ourselves in the storm raised the A team's credibility with the command staff more than anything else we had done professionally prior to that. Team sections were designated for specific rotations by days on call, and we slept in the minimal-care tent over night—hoping that no casualties would arrive.

Midmorning on February 27, word came around that casualties were likely to arrive within several hours. The first section prepared to receive any combat stress casualties by getting to know the hospital staff on duty and informing them of our mission. The remainder of the team set up the sleeping tents for the next several days. When casualties started arriving in midafternoon, all non first-section personnel (except those on guard detail) were available to help with patient flow—in a variety of locations—as litter bearers, riding with the ground ambulance crews out to the helicopters, and working with the division liaison NCOs.

The first section floated in the minimal-care area, talking with incoming wounded soldiers, preop, postop, and in the holding area while waiting for evacuation to the next echelon of care. It was by talking with these wounded soldiers that the maxim of "treating all wounded soldiers as potential combat stress casualties" was proved true. Giving these soldiers a chance to talk about their battlefield experiences leading up to being wounded, and their reactions to it, appeared to be very beneficial for them. Most of the other medical personnel were focused on triage and not on soldier reactions to their recent traumas. There seemed to be a lessening of tension as the soldiers went through impromptu debriefing—especially when talking about the death of fellow soldiers or riding in a helicopter with a dead soldier from their unit. The unit chaplains were also of invaluable help (as they had an established entry into the hospital when A team members were still viewed somewhat suspiciously as outsiders) in identifying soldiers and/or staff at risk.

The first identified combat stress casualty came in on the first evening. He was identified in the triage area by ER staff as appearing unresponsive and having difficulty hearing and concentrating beyond what could be explained from his blast injury. He had an essentially normal physical examination and gave vague details on his injury. After referral to the combat stress casualty tent, he was entered in the program with a diagnosis of mild to moderate combat stress reaction. His debriefing revealed that he and his squad mate were truck drivers and that his codriver had picked up some cluster bomb units. Evidently, the vibration of the truck on the roads caused the bomblets to explode in the cab, killing the driver and exposing the patient in the passenger seat to possible injury and subsequently extreme sleep deprivation. After the debriefing, a Meal Ready to Eat (MRE), and cleaning up, he slept overnight in the combat stress casualty tent. The content of the debriefing was his reaction to the death of the other soldier in part due to their ignorance of the potential danger of the bomblets. In the morning he was ready to return to duty, but there was no system set up for his return. The theater had not matured enough to allow division and corps personnel officers to establish opportunities for return to duty in one's own unit. Supply trains were also not yet established, so that potential avenue of return to duty was not available. While waiting for his return to duty to be effected, a second debriefing was initiated during which the soldier was outnumbered five to one (three section members, one chaplain, and one chaplain's assistant). He eventually was airevacuated back on the third hospital day when orders came to reduce the hospital census and no means had been established to return him to duty with local assets.

The second section was on call on the second day, and they continued the floating procedures established on day one—circulating through the minimal-care areas, triage, emergency room, and intensive care wards, talking with casualties and hospital staff. Their ability to circulate was hampered by the posting of guards by one hospital to control access to those who had a need to be present (A team members were not granted entry, as they were not recognized as part of the task force which had a legitimate need to have access to patients and hospital staff as part of their combat stress control mission. This hospital was the one that A team had not had a chance to establish a working relationship with).

High-stress sections of the hospitals were identified for stress debriefings to be given over the next several days (ER, Lab, OR). A soldier with unusual gastrointestinal symptoms was referred to the on-call section as a potential combat stress casualty with conversion disorder. He responded eagerly to the interventions, both medical (intravenous hydration and bowel rest) and psychiatric (rest reassurance and talking/debriefing). After some validation that his symptoms were responding to medication and reassurance that his feelings of fear, distrust, and isolation were normal and expectable reactions to the abnormal situation of being in a combat environment, he was ready to return to duty after less than 24 hours. (His unit was located several miles away, so he was able to be returned to his unit without problems.)

By the second day, casualties were primarily Iraqi prisoners of war or civilians. More attention focused on the needs of the task force personnel. Debriefings of several sections were conducted with the hospital at which we had a prior working relationship. Efforts to present our services to the other hospital were rebuffed. Other circumstances that hampered task force debriefings were rumor control and the orders to dismantle most of the hospital (except for the forward surgical element) for deployment back to Saudi Arabia.

Once back in Saudi Arabia, the OM team reconstituted in one location for the first time since early November 1990. Much of the command elements were focused on administrative details associated with redeployment: after-action reports, chronological summaries, evaluation reports, award submissions, and movement planning. The debriefing mission of the OM team was delegated to a lower priority. Attempts were made to debrief an engineer company which had suffered heavy losses only to discover it had already been debriefed by one of the psychiatrists from an evacuation hospital. Other units were not contacted due to lack of knowledge of their locations and no prior working relationships.

The unit redeployed to Fort Benning on April 19, 1991.

SUMMARY

Be flexible and drink plenty of water were good words to live by. All psychiatrists (and other mental health personnel) need to know combat psychiatry—not just military psychiatry (medical evaluation boards and chapter discharges, Army Drug and Alcohol Prevention and Consultation Program [ADAPCP], sanity boards, compassionate reassignment letters, etc.). Combat psychiatry is conducted in a field environment and is not office based. The primary missions are education, consultation, and prevention of combat stress casualties. Preexisting relationships are much better than showing up at the last minute, especially with other medical units. Only one person in the unit was selected for his specific skills. He was the commander. We did well, but that was due to our flexibility and can-do attitude, not because of our selection for combat skills.

These types of units need more practice working together before mobilization. Earlier deployment would also allow for working relationships to develop with both medical and corps support units. Later redeployment would allow for more unit debriefings and reunification work.

Mental health professionals and paraprofessionals need to know how the Army is organized for combat and how various elements function, who has inherent medical support, and who does not. Awareness of maintenance and supply echelons is important. The OM team needs more nonmedical MOSs— supply, maintenance, communications, and field sanitation. Book knowledge and prior experience (West Point, Reserve Officer Training Corps, and the Uniform Services University of the Health Services) were very helpful but no substitute for field practice. We need to practice in garrison as we fight in war. More stringent predeployment screening of personnel is important.

It is hoped that the lessons learned in the Persian Gulf War will make future deployment of combat stress control teams easier and more productive.

6

Combat Psychiatry in the 1st Armored Division

Loree Sutton and Daniel W. Clark

INTRODUCTION

This chapter is an account of the challenges encountered by the mental health team of the 1st Armored Division from the time the division was notified for deployment to the Gulf War to the division's eventual homecoming after the war. The division had expected to be inactivated within a year, but on November 9, 1990 the division was directed to prepare to deploy to the Gulf War. At the time of deployment announcement, the 1st Armored Division's mental health team consisted of one psychiatrist, one pregnant social worker, and four behavioral science specialists, two of whom were new to the Army and still inprocessing from their basic and advanced individual training (a soldier's entry level training). Deploying for war would be their first real field exercise.

To fill the critical positions with experienced personnel, the mental health team submitted a roster through the military personnel system identifying experienced mental health personnel available in Germany who were eager and ready to join this team. No orders were forthcoming (with the exception of the division psychologist, who finally received orders the week prior to departure). The 1st Armored Division mental health team deployed to the Gulf with half of the team members without prior division mental health experience, while coveted veteran mental health personnel chomped at their bits, still tethered to their hospital positions in Germany.

The mental health team sought to become players in the division. Everyone took their mental health job seriously—respecting rules, training for clinical and field skill improvement, inviting criticism, assuming the best about others' intentions, and nurturing bonds of loyalty which transcend any personal idiosyncrasy. Team members reached out to shake hands, talk shop, and drink bad coffee all over the division, and they shivered in the snow during field training.

Team members even photocopied and collated more than 5000 copies of training materials for two a day team building workshops conducted in collaboration with unit ministry teams.

PREDEPLOYMENT

Through a combination of bartering and luck, the team obtained the tents, cots, and heaters needed to achieve its combat mission. Getting vehicles presented more of a challenge. Vehicles were not obtained until the team was in Saudi Arabia and only because training/consultation services demanded the team's presence among the division's many units. This surge in demand ultimately resulted in the division supplying two of the three vehicles authorized for the team.

To support commanders by screening soldiers for deployment, the team made a working assumption that any soldier able to draw a paycheck every month is able to go to war. With this attitude, it became possible to deal with the rush of combat inspired maladies in a straightforward manner. Soldiers disabled by legitimate medical or psychiatric problems were referred for medical board separation. Alleged pregnancies were confirmed by blood tests. Soldiers with alcohol problems were enrolled in the "Track IV" and deployed to Saudi Arabia. (The Army's alcohol rehabilitation program has three levels, or tracks, that make up the overall treatment program. Track IV allows for deployment, with follow up care provided by mental health personnel in the combat theater.) Soldiers applying for conscientious objector status completed their applications and deployed for full duty pending response from the Department of the Army. Soldiers experiencing "gas mask phobia" were checked for proper fit and given intensive breathing focus training exercises. Soldiers breaking the rules were disciplined accordingly.

To assure that distressed soldiers would be treated as far forward as possible, mental health team members trained commanders, command sergeants major, first sergeants, junior unit leaders, doctors, physician assistants, and unit ministry teams in recognizing, treating, and preventing battle fatigue casualties. Front loading the system with this forward expertise freed the mental health team members to devote more time to complex clinical problems, follow up training, and consultation. Unit chaplains agreed to serve as the first link in the chain of referral for managing soldiers in distress. This role was a natural extension of what chaplains already do in ministering to the fear and concerns of their soldiers. The commanding general approved this policy, and it was published in the division operations order.

As the team attempted to mobilize the division's communities and family members to move from shock and denial into effective support and action, team members had to remind themselves to heed their own training messages on surviving extraordinary stress. Members of the team recognized that they were not exempt from experiencing the full emotional stress of this deployment and war, and they had to strengthen themselves if they were to help others. Predeployment stressors included hearing ghastly casualty estimates, choking through an endless series of goodbyes with loved ones, missing holiday festivities, writing the "last letter," and raging at all that was beyond our knowing or control. Throughout the deployment, team leaders brainstormed ways of coping with what might lie ahead —anticipating feelings of guilt, despair, and helplessness; role playing the agonizing triage process of deciding who gets treated and who must wait (or even die); and acknowledging the power of looking out for and leaning on each other.

DEPLOYMENT

To provide rest and recovery for soldiers requiring one to three days of treatment, the team attached two pairs of behavioral science specialists and the division social worker to circuit ride between the three forward brigade medical companies, leaving the division psychiatrist, psychologist, and one pair of behavioral science specialists in the main medical company. During the trek into Iraq, soldiers not responding to unit support and panic—buster breathing techniques would be referred for medication induced sleep therapy and kept within the combat support area—there was no turning back at this point. Doctors and physician assistants carried a Benadryl, Haldol, Thorazine, and Valium for use as needed. Fortunately, these medications were generally not needed.

Prior to moving to the forward assembly area just south of the Iraqi border, the team collocated with a 20 bed psychiatric unit of an evacuation hospital.   This unit's senior psychiatrist was from one of the Army hospitals in Germany, and she was well known to the division psychiatrist. This hospital psychiatrist's clinical savvy and buoyant spirit allowed division soldiers, and often mental health team members, to return to effective duty following a brief visit to her unit.

Prior to deployment, team members provided the division physicians and physician assistants with training in the treatment of combat stress casualties and coping with wounded enemy soldiers, civilians, and children. Although the team addressed the difficulty in treating enemy and civilian injuries, the scope of this challenge surpassed any of the team's advance planning. The most valuable component of this training may have been to encourage a mind set which anticipated the unexpected. Providing ongoing support to medical personnel became one of the major activities following the ground war. Memories of starving families and children maimed by cluster bombs remain indelibly etched in the minds of team members.

Requests from commanders to "fix or get rid" of problem soldiers posed a difficult challenge whose importance cannot be underestimated. Spiraling into a power struggle with a commander who knows his soldier is "crazy" and cannot understand how the mental health team can possibly clear him or her psychiatrically makes everyone a loser. Mental health professionals and commanders must work together to find the best solution, recognizing that clearing a soldier psychiatrically frees the commander to take whatever action is deemed necessary, usually disciplinary, knowing that the soldier's behavior did not result from a psychiatric disorder. Working constructively with commanders is critical for maintaining the team's professional credibility as well as for sending a no nonsense message to soldiers that they will be held accountable for their behavior. If acting "crazy" is the ticket home, a division rapidly becomes a hotbed for "wanna be psychos."

Passing messages between mental health team members spread out at different locations was usually very difficult. Messages sent through the main support battalion often did not survive the journey to the medical company. The most reliable means of contacting other team members was sending messages via the senior unit commanders to the division psychiatrist who attended the daily division command briefing. Contacting the mental health team members attached in forward units was similarly unpredictable unless someone actually drove directly to their locations.

The mental health team encouraged unit commanders to use the cease-fire time for debriefing combat experiences by giving them a refresher course in facilitating this healing work. Team members conducted site visits to units exposed to the most intense fighting and provided follow up support to medical personnel coping with the horrors of human "collateral damage." During the weeks following the cease-fire, team members witnessed a startling pattern of daredevil behavior which resulted in deaths for no reason. This behavior included collecting explosive devices as souvenirs. The team speculated on the psychological underpinnings fueling this behavior and developed a briefing for commanders on what the team termed "cease-fire let down." This innovative contribution helped team members and commanders work together to curb further tragedy.

REDEPLOYMENT

The 1st Armored Division established Camp Kasserine adjacent to King Khalid Military City, Saudi Arabia, to help division soldiers make a healthy transition back to peacetime living. The camp included a post exchange [PX], shaded patio seating, a stage for live entertainment, a multivideo theater, commercial phones, a pool hall, a video game arcade, basketball courts, fast food (free burgers, fries, and drinks), a museum displaying tanks captured in battle, a post office, laundry service, and a sleeping bag exchange. A one stop business center had personnel, reenlistment, legal, medical, mental health, Red Cross, inspector general, and finance services. This garrison atmosphere helped soldiers take the first step in winding down from the rush and intensity of life on the battlefield. Team members again linked up with the unit ministry teams in command consultation and outreach efforts.

LESSONS AND RECOMMENDATIONS

The following lessons and recommendations were gleaned from our Gulf War experience:

Collocate forward team members with brigade unit ministry teams.

Position elements of corps-level mental health OM teams with division main medical companies as soon as possible following notice of deployment.

Train and formally identify chaplains to serve as the first point of contact for all stress related referrals.

Identify experienced mental health team members in advance to fill division vacancies in the event of combat—personnel managers must target experience as a first priority (sending untrained and unprepared fledglings to war as mental health experts is unconscionable).

Trust doctrine, yet stay flexible and creative. Reinforce the expectation at all levels that even severely distressed soldiers can recover for full duty—the most extreme emotional reactions must be treated as normal responses to the abnormal setting of combat.

Work to earn the respect of senior division leaders—their support is imperative for fulfilling the mental health mission.

Never underestimate the power of sleep, water, food, hygiene, and local support.

Be prepared to manage cot wetting, suicide aftermath, "gas mask" phobia, recovering "12 steppers," recent and delayed effects of trauma, and existential questions emerging in the face of potential death.

Adapt record keeping procedures to reflect the Spartan nature of the combat environment—lack of files, secure storage space, copy machines, computers, or appointments.

Streamline intake and evaluation procedures in anticipation of mass casualty scenarios—given 200 medical casualties per hour (the initial estimate by theater planners), we expected at least 50 stress related cases per hour (the "50 minute hour" in garrison gives way to the "50 second hour" in combat).

The combat mental health "bag of tricks" must include modules on battle fatigue, stress management, cease-fire, and homecoming reunion.

Target division leaders for training in all these areas—if leaders have the tools they need, soldiers will benefit.

Finally, relationships are the key to surviving and thriving in a division during peacetime, and they are a critical necessity during combat. Close working ties with commanders, staffers, and senior noncommissioned officers comprise the foundation underlying all that we do.

7

Combat Psychiatry the "First Team" Way: First Cavalry Division Mental Health Operations during the Persian Gulf War

Spencer J. Campbell and Charles C. Engel, Jr.

INTRODUCTION

On the morning of August 10, 1990, the routine training schedule of the 1st Cavalry Division was interrupted: The "First Team" was on tactical alert for overseas deployment. In the weeks that followed, a sense of anxious uncertainty prevailed in the community surrounding our garrison home of Fort Hood, Texas. Newly painted desert camouflage vehicles were a ubiquitous reminder to soldiers, their families, and the community that we were preparing for war. In the division mental health team, we were facing the daunting challenge of providing overseas and perhaps combat mental health support to an armored division of approximately 17,000 soldiers. Prominent in our minds was the possible worst case of combat stress casualties exceeding the numbers wounded and killed in action.

We have written this chapter to describe some of the key challenges the 1st Cavalry Division Mental Health Section faced and how we responded to them. The principles on which our responses were based can be summarized as six C's: soldier, section, and mission Credibility; operational and logistical Cohesion; Combat stress prevention; Centralization of clinical services; forward deployed Contact teams; and Critical event stress debriefings. Several significant emotional events illustrate how these principles helped us.

COMBAT PSYCHIATRY IN "THE CAV": SIX C's

The C's are listed in the order of their relative importance to successful completion of the division mental health mission.

Credibility

Much is said in the combat psychiatric literature about how to treat combat stress and battle fatigue, but little is said about the importance of credibility on making treatment plans happen. Loss or maintenance of credibility takes place on several levels and, in our view, always makes or breaks an organization's ability to be effective. Credibility starts at the individual soldier level, but must be developed at the section and mission levels as well. At the individual level, division mental health personnel, including officers, must learn to "walk the walk, and talk the talk." In other words, to be seen as an insider in the division, mental health personnel must at a minimum respect the formal and informal rules of military bearing and etiquette, be practiced in essential field skills, and exercise careful judgment around clinical issues. This sounds obvious, but the first two points may involve homework and personal assistance from others with more proficiency in soldier skills. This is time well spent, however, since there is no quicker way to lose the trust and respect of your team and division than to appear cavalier or uninformed about allegedly simple soldierly matters.

Similarly, to build section credibility, the division mental health team must manifest cohesiveness and actively pursue its mission. Most commanders and soldiers know little about the division mental health section (DMHS) mission. In most cases, they will learn the mission from watching and listening to members of the DMHS. For example, a commander may have doubts about offering the mental health team vehicles if he or she does not see the team pursuing an active forward mission that requires mobility. Early and often during the deployment, we sent mental health contact teams to maneuver battalions offering clinical services and preventive briefings. We think this demonstration of a mobile mental health mission figured prominently in our ability to keep three vehicles throughout the deployment.

Mission credibility is especially important. Soldiers frequently view the mental health mission with a mixture of suspicion, stigma, and fear of career damage. Mental health personnel must spend time with soldiers in nonclinical settings (e.g., preventive briefings, training activities, and unit functions) to reduce concerns based on these negative stereotypes.

Cohesion

Cohesion is important to team effectiveness and credibility. We distinguish two overlapping types of cohesion, which we call operational and logistical cohesion. Operational cohesion involves the interpersonal ties and command quality that occurs within a hierarchical unit pursuing a single common mission. This is contrasted to logistical cohesion, which involves similar ties between personnel from elements with slightly different missions, who must rely on one another to move in a tactical or combat environment. For example, during the

Gulf War, units developed forward area support teams (FASTs). These were unit subelements designed to leave quickly on the initiation of a ground movement. Prior to combat, FASTs were often located one or two hundred meters from the main element, allowing them to develop a sense of their own equipment, transportation, personnel, supply, and other needs. Cohesion among FAST participants can be viewed as a form of logistical cohesion. To be fully effective, the division mental health team must develop cohesion with elements within its own division, battalion, and medical company (logistical cohesion) as well as within its own organization (operational cohesion).

Combat Stress Prevention

There are several reasons that combat stress prevention is important. Not all of them directly relate to preventing combat stress. Preventive briefings present ideal opportunities to establish credibility and build cohesion. During preventive activities, section soldiers are visible, work together, and actively pursue the mission. Preventive briefings may help identify motivated soldiers in need of brief supportive assistance who might otherwise avoid clinical care. Often, when we briefed units on preventive measures, soldiers would engage us privately in short discussions of personal, family, or other problems. These soldiers seemingly had few hidden agendas and were generally motivated to implement the self-help strategies we gave them. Most told us they would not have come to see us if we had not come to their unit.

Centralized Clinical Services

Perhaps the most essential combat mental health team role is that of the division's mental health services gatekeeper. Ideally, stress casualties are evaluated by the mental health team before accessing higher echelons of theater health care. This, of course, is because the farther psychiatrically disabled soldiers get from their unit, the poorer their prognosis will be as gain increases and the psychological bonds between soldier and unit fragment. Centralization of clinical services enhances ability to collect reliable, population based data. Thus, data on service utilization among division soldiers can be gathered, and the division can better account for soldiers in the combat mental health system.

Forward Deployed Contact Teams

We used the division mental health team contact teams to meet the requirement for forward, centralized combat mental health services. A dilemma for us was deciding the appropriate balance between centralization and forward treatment. If we sacrificed forward treatment for centralization, we might have fielded a single large section at the division-level medical company. If we sacrificed centralization for forward treatment, we might have placed a single mental health team member at nearly all of the maneuver battalion medical platoons. Cohesion was also a consideration. The more centralized we were, the greater the opportunity for developing sound operational cohesion. Conversely, the farther forward we were, the greater the importance of logistical cohesion. Since smaller forward deployed mental health team elements would not be formally assigned to collocating units, more effort would be required to develop relationships with members of the collocating unit. These relationships might later translate into mutual commitment during combat crises.

The balance we struck was to place contact teams at each of the three brigade-level medical companies and a fourth at the division-level medical company. We deployed with a psychiatrist, social work officer, psychologist, the enlisted section NonCommissioned officer in charge (NCOIC), and five other enlisted behavioral science specialists (91Gs). Each contact team consisted of an officer (one was led by the NCOIC) and one or two 91Gs. The psychiatrist and two 91Gs worked with the division level medical company. The other teams collocated with the brigade-level medical companies. Each of the forward teams had its own vehicle, basic equipment, and tent.

Two observations on the logistical cohesion problem mentioned earlier are worth noting. First, the decision to use contact teams should be made as early as possible. Forward deployed teams rely on collocated units for essentials such as food, ammunition, and vehicle maintenance. Lack of logistical cohesion between a contact team and its collocating medical company can endanger the forward mental health mission and even threaten the lives of contact team members during a crisis. Second, careful thought must be given to the composition of each team. We kept our two most junior 91Gs at the division level in the belief that maximizing rank, military leadership experience, and credibility would enhance forward teams' ability to develop and maintain adequate logistical cohesion. Indeed, our entire decision to use forward deployed contact teams was made easier by the fact that our social worker and psychologist had prior enlisted experience and the latter also had Vietnam combat experience. Our NCOIC was a former school teacher and college athlete who was respected by all.

Critical Event Stress Debriefings (CESDs)

When doing a CESD in response to a crisis, the response team takes the following steps: Establish communication with commanders of affected units; determine the circle of crisis impact, to include victims, witnesses, rescuers, friends, and members of affected units; convene the affected groups for information, education, sharing, referral, and normalization; counsel/assess individuals; and reevaluate and follow up. The vignettes that follow show that some of our most powerful experiences as combat mental health care providers came while participating in CESDs.

ILLUSTRATING THE PRINCIPALS: FOCUS ON FIVE SIGNIFICANT EMOTIONAL EVENTS

The following vignettes capture a few of our more important and lasting memories of the Gulf War. Combat mental health practice is markedly different from hospital-based practice. Our primary goals in this section are to describe difficult situations that can arise during combat deployment and to illustrate how the six C's helped us accomplish our mission.

Event One: An Effort at Prevention

The first major opportunity we faced came shortly after the alert while we were still at Fort Hood. Once we learned of the deployment, we decided that a major predeployment combat stress prevention campaign was necessary to achieve section credibility and combat stress prevention.

Each member of the division was required to go through nuclear biological chemical (NBC) refresher training, and the division surgeon approved combat stress control briefing stations at each of two tear gas chambers. We opted to rotate a 91G at each station, with one officer supervising the two chambers. Briefing teams and soldiers all wore chemical protective gear while on site, and the hours were long, beginning in morning darkness and often extending past dusk. Soldiers would generally arrive in groups of 10 to 25 sometimes before and other times after entering the chamber.

It was August in central Texas, and the temperatures hovered consistently in the 95- to 105-degree range, making adequate hydration difficult and MOPP gear extremely uncomfortable. The actual combat stress briefing took no longer than about 10 minutes. Its focus changed slightly depending on the general rank and position of the audience. A brief didactic portion covered the signs and symptoms of combat stress, the buddy system of monitoring for early signs, leadership issues, and proper battlefield treatment, hygiene, and prevention. We also gave information regarding where division mental health team assets would be located in the theater of operations, adding that in the majority of cases, combat stress and subsequent battle fatigue could be prevented or recognized and treated without mental health assistance. In closing the briefing, we did a role-play on the importance and technique of disarming a disoriented combat stress casualty. As soldiers passed through our station, many wondered aloud whether Iraq would use chemical weapons. Television images of chemically burned Kurds provided these soldiers with all the motivation they needed to take this exercise seriously.

Eventually, we got to know the soldiers on the NBC team, and a few times division mental health team members were entrusted to escort personnel from the four medical companies through the chamber. If soldiers panicked in the chamber, mental health team members would assist them and eventually escort them back through the chamber.

The NBC team's goal was to ensure that each soldier developed confidence in their chemical equipment. Similarly, we felt that by being available to soldiers at the gas chamber, we could bolster their confidence in their division mental health team. Ultimately, we provided preventive briefings to over 12,000 soldiers.

This combat stress prevention campaign was the first of several preventive efforts we mounted. It proved essential as a rapid way of achieving early mission, section, and individual credibility and operational and logistical cohesion. Although we used the NBC training site as the place for our briefings, the weapons training site might have been another opportunity to catch the majority of soldiers in a unit as part of a predeployment train up.

These briefings, and the early visibility they provided, served to introduce us to division soldiers; demystify our mission, create opportunities for us to interface with company, battalion, brigade, and division command; and develop important attachments within our section and between our section and the division. We were surprised by the number of soldiers who did not know the division had intrinsic mental health assets.

Overseas, many soldiers remembered us from these and other preventive briefings and struck up conversations with us. This would later help us maintain a sense of division morale and served as a measure of our rapport within the division.

Several key general and field-grade officers attended these predeployment briefings. Instant credibility was gained with a new division surgeon, who worked closely with us to arrange the briefings. Subsequent access to maneuver battalions was eased in some cases because commanders came to view us as knowledgeable about the combat mission. Indeed, we were most flattered by the comment from one brigade commander: "Most docs wear the Class B [garrison] uniform and live in distant offices with little green plants in them and stuff. You guys aren't like that, are you?"

We noted that soldiers enjoy participating during briefings. A technique we used with good success was role-playing. For the predeployment briefings, we used role-play to demonstrate how to disarm a disoriented soldier. In other briefings, role-play worked nicely to demonstrate points about relationships between NCOs and officers and returning home to family and friends after combat. In a death and dying briefing, we had senior NCOs and officers write their own obituaries as well as mock letters to the imaginary families of soldiers killed in action. This approach was well received and helped to create relationships between soldiers within units and between Division Mental Health Staff [DMHS] staff and units' soldiers.

Event Two: The Christmas of Our Discontents

Christmas of 1990 found the First Team preparing for movement toward the Iraqi border. The January 15 deadline had been set for Iraq to withdraw from Kuwait, and the rhetoric was flowing freely from Baghdad. Most soldiers were of the opinion that we were preparing to engage Iraq in ground combat. Everyone was working long hours, the sand storms were more severe, and the holiday mood was decidedly somber.

At about 2200 hours on Christmas eve, the medical company commander came to our tent for assistance. He explained, to our disbelief, that an entire supply platoon had come to sick call with a variety of vague and medically unsubstantiated physical complaints. He asked if there was anything we could do to sort out the situation and return these soldiers to their duties.

First, we met with the sick-call physicians. All agreed that this angry group of soldiers was protesting something. The platoon sergeant, platoon leader, and first sergeant appeared a bit confused and expressed shock at their soldiers' behavior. They indicated that these soldiers were normally high functioning and hard working. Even though the company had been working long hours prepositioning supplies to the north, neither company nor platoon leadership had noticed any problems. They had been preparing to convoy that night when their soldiers started to complain of physical symptoms.

We gathered ourselves and decided on a way to approach the platoon. Our social worker and psychologist would do a "good cop–bad cop" intervention that we hoped would gain the soldiers' attention and then catalyze negotiation of a solution between the soldiers and their command. We informed the unit's command of the plan, and with their consent we proceeded. Everyone joined the platoon in the holding area. First, the social worker (a former enlisted marine who can still play the part) read the soldiers their rights. He then told them they had each received a full medical evaluation for their complaints and no medical problems had been found. They were therefore in violation of the Uniformed Code of Military Justice by portraying themselves as ill. This, they were informed, could lead to court marshals, dishonorable discharges, or even prison terms. There was a stir, and the soldiers' eyes got big as they began to realize the gravity of their actions. A couple of soldiers began to make excuses for their behavior. One sergeant finally said, "I don't think it's fair for us to have to work on Christmas." It appeared we had landed the real problem.

The psychologist then spoke on behalf of the soldiers. "Doc, these seem like reasonable soldiers who've just made an error in judgment. Let me talk with them and see if something can't be worked out." The level of tension dropped, and everyone but the psychologist and the platoon and its leaders left the tent so they could discuss their differences privately. The psychologist learned that no one had explained to the soldiers why they had to work on Christmas. They did not realize that most division soldiers would be working that day. The platoon leader and sergeant explained what they knew of the division's plan to move north soon after Christmas. Eventually, it was agreed that the soldiers could work hard and efficiently if they knew the platoon leadership would find time off for them as soon as possible. The first sergeant agreed to ensure that this promise was kept. The psychologist added some final words for both soldiers and leaders on the unit communication and appropriate use of the chain of command for communication purposes. Shortly after midnight, the platoon returned to the work site. Later, visits to the unit convinced us that the platoon's difficulties were largely resolved and that the unit was functioning normally.

We offer this vignette as an example of some of the unusual clinical and organizational problems mental health teams may be faced with in a tactical environment. The psychologist and social worker acted essentially as a crisis response team to a critical event. Their intervention contains some of the basic elements of a CESD. They established communication with platoon leaders. Failure to consult with "management" might have resulted in an ill-conceived intervention that would be undone later in the absence of an outside consultant. They convened the affected groups—namely, the platoon and its leaders—and initiated an imaginative intervention leading to a clear organizational diagnosis. Sharing of information and the successful mediation and negotiation of a normalizing work agreement soon followed. Adequate follow up was obtained through the use of both DMHS and battalion chaplain visits. Centralization of our services made it easy for medical staff to consult us and allowed us to gather mental health service utilization data. Such information can yield early clues to organizational relapse.

Events Three and Four: Busting the Berm

One of our brigade contact teams supported several reconnaissance, or "berm buster," missions in the days just prior to the start of the Gulf War ground combat. These missions involved movement of armored battalions beyond the massive sand berm that Iraq had placed along its southern border. During these operations, the division suffered four soldiers killed and 12 wounded in action. The next two vignettes are accounts of CESDs done after the contact team provided forward medical treatment for soldiers wounded in these operations.

The 91G and I approached the M113 Air Defense track that had taken a direct hit and lost two crew members. We found the crew inventorying their equipment and were both immediately overwhelmed by the soldiers' heightened emotions. I spoke to a soldier standing on top of the track and saw that he was close to tears. I asked him if he had heard any news of his sergeant, who had been evacuated with second- and third-degree burns. When he said he had not, we told him the story of how we had helped treat him shortly after he was wounded. We told him he was conscious and had spoken with us prior to being evacuated; he was in a lot of pain, not likely to return soon, but sure to recover. This news appeared to make him feel better. We asked if we could help him and the crew with their inventory, and he invited us to climb on board.

Once on the track, we could see that its top part had been blown off in the battle. The soldier described to us how one sergeant had taken a direct hit from an artillery or mortar round and been decapitated. Another, the one we had helped, had been burned by the explosion because he was standing below where the first soldier was killed. He vividly described how the decapitated sergeant's lower body had fallen into the track and settled to the floor for the rest of the crew to see. The other crew members also began to talk us through their combat experience while they continued to remove the ammunition and equipment from the track. One soldier got angry and started to cry. He held out his hand and showed us pieces of skin and bone. "This is all that's left of my sergeant," he said.

We remained with these soldiers until they completed their inventory. We talked with the crew about returning to combat. All three of those remaining had less than three years in the Army. Two said it was important for them to go into Iraq. One said he wanted to be placed in a support position but remain with his unit even if it returned to combat. Eventually the first two soldiers stayed in their jobs and the third drove a fuel truck for his unit. All performed well during the ground campaign. All three received awards for outstanding combat service.

The second debriefing involved a Bradley scout crew that had also been hit in the same battle as the Air Defense track. We met with the survivors and walked with them to the motor pool where their Bradley (an armored personnel carrier) had been towed. I asked the crew to describe what had occurred. A staff sergeant immediately crouched to the ground and used a stick in the sand to diagram the battle. His speech was rapid as he related how the track commander of another Bradley had been hit and killed with a round. "I remember it like slow motion. It's just so unreal," he said. He told of watching the same Bradley take three more direct hits. Almost without thinking, he and his crew had then left their Bradley while under fire, moved to the hit Bradley, and started doing first aid. One of the sergeant's crew ran to a wounded soldier and initiated medical aid. As the rounds came closer, the crewman covered the wounded soldier with his body, taking a fatal head wound as a result. The staff sergeant became visibly angry as he told of going to his Bradley, positioning it behind the disabled Bradley, loading a round, locating the Iraqi position, and "terminating" it. Ground ambulance crews then arrived and stabilized and evacuated the wounded. Iraqi fire then started to focus on other locations.

We shifted the focus to the other crew members for their comments. The staff sergeant continued on with pressured speech and started to go through the battle again. The 91G took the sergeant aside, and the debriefing continued with the remaining crew members. These soldiers concurred with the sergeant's account of the battle. Some crew members said that they had blocked out many of the details, and the sergeant's description had brought them back. We opened the Bradley and saw its partially charred interior. The mood was like a wake.

These soldiers knew that we had assisted their wounded and handled their dead. They asked about "the L Tee" (their lieutenant and platoon leader) who had been burned about the face, taken some shrapnel, and injured his back in the battle. I told them what I knew—that he was awake, talking, and in a lot of pain when he was loaded on the evacuation helicopter. He seemed okay, but probably would not return to the unit soon if at all.

These crew members were later assigned to other crews. We visited them prior to their next battle, and they had spray painted "We're Back" on the outside of their new Bradley. They all served well in the ground war, and three Silver Stars were awarded to involved soldiers, one posthumously.

These powerful vignettes offer striking testimony to several principles. An outstanding feature of both CESDs is the quick rapport achieved by the forward deployed contact team with the crew members. In general, combat veterans' level of suspicion toward the "strangers" was in direct proportion to the person's distance from combat. The contact team had positioned itself centrally so they could be aware of the status of casualties and even participate in their medical care. Consequently, an implicit bond existed that was based on a mutual combat experience. Thus, the contact team was almost immediately trusted by both of these track crews.

This team was easily our most active both prior to and during the ground attack. They had assumed a very high profile among the maneuver elements in their brigade through the use of stress prevention briefings and regular attendance at command and staff meetings. We feel strongly that the level of credibility and logistical cohesion developed in this process was essential to their success. These "berm buster" operations were highly sensitive and dangerous. If the contact team was not viewed as combat ready, its presence on the forward deployed medical team would never have been allowed.

Event Five: Death in the Division Area

Even during staging operations, a combat division becomes surprisingly extended. Indeed, during the initial overseas deployment, the division had soldiers and equipment located in the states, the port of Dammam, Saudi Arabia, and 200 kilometers northwest in the middle of the Saudi desert. As the following vignette shows, mental health services may be required at the times and places where you least expect it.

A false sense of security and an almost festive mood had evolved as we had quickly moved north past the berm and far into Iraq, seemingly unopposed. Then the news: Three battalion soldiers had just been killed and one wounded in an accident involving unexploded ordnance. When the convoy halted for the night, the two 91Gs went to see what they could learn about the incident while I went to the battalion command post (CP). Soldiers were shifting nervously outside their vehicles while talking quietly. At the CP, some officers were cursing the soldiers' stupidity for "playing with" the ordnance. Some expressed relief that these were not their soldiers. All the soldiers killed were from the ordnance company. The ordnance company commander, normally tough and strack, was standing quietly to the side. The unit's Executive Officer [XO] stood next to her looking a little shocked. There was generally a lot of head hanging and foot shuffling.

The battalion commander was planning an ad hoc command and staff meeting. As part of the meeting, I was to brief the commanders on how they should address their units about the soldiers' deaths. The assistant division and battalion chaplains were with us, and we agreed to work together. The bodies of the dead soldiers were brought by ambulance to the campsite and loaded into a graves registration van. The wounded soldier was evacuated by helicopter. Soldiers pushed to get close and see something as the bodies were loaded. Doctors and medics had to work to keep curious soldiers away.

The 91Gs had learned that the crew members from three chemical company tracks helping to guard our perimeter had witnessed the accident. The two chaplains and I convened the three track crews, a total of around 15 soldiers, and debriefed them together. We asked them to describe what they had seen. A sergeant said, "I couldn't believe it. There were cluster bombs all around, and these guys got off the road, two PFCs [Private First Class] jumped out and one dude started pickin' 'em up! I saw that and I put my head in the track. I wasn't havin' anything to do with that!" A staff sergeant told us he saw one of the PFCs picking up ordnance and the second close behind. A sergeant, he informed us, had followed them out of their Hum Vee looking very unsure and slowly walked toward the PFCs. The first PFC picked up some ordnance, inspected it, and turned to hand it to the other PFC just as the sergeant walked up. Another staff sergeant chimed in and told us he had hollered at them to put the ordnance down. Then the first PFC looked up with a funny smile as if embarrassed, and the bomb detonated as he was handing it to the second PFC, immediately killing all three soldiers. Nobody had even seen the wounded soldier, but there was speculation that he was still in the Hum Vee. We shifted the conversation to the other crew members. No one had known the soldiers personally. "I can't believe it! The war's over and these guys go and get themselves killed," said one soldier. Another sergeant expressed disgust that an NCO could show such bad judgment. We discussed common symptoms people have normally after witnessing disasters and gave advice on appropriate resources they could seek if they wanted further counseling or mental health assistance. The assistant division chaplain closed the meeting with a word of prayer for the soldiers who had died, their families back home, the division, and our FAST.

While addressing the command and staff meeting, I learned from commanders that the sergeant who was killed was popular in his unit. Few soldiers had known the other two soldiers, since they had both arrived at the unit in the weeks just prior to combat. It appeared that no one else had witnessed the accident. I advised the command to stay with "normal" routine as much as possible. I suggested they use the event as a reminder to their units that danger was everywhere and that we must not let down our guards, even if it appeared the conflict was over. I again addressed common signs and symptoms following disasters and encouraged commanders to remain sensitive to soldiers' needs. The theme of the meeting was to "get over it," so I suggested that commanders avoid prematurely extinguishing discussion of the deaths. Thinking of the ordnance commander, I offered to speak privately with anyone to address questions. We offered to meet with whole units as requested. Before the process was complete, we talked with the ordnance company, several of the deceased sergeant's friends, his section, and the medics who had recovered the soldiers' bodies. I personally offered the ordnance supply commander the opportunity to talk privately, but she declined. She felt her unit could manage the situation internally, a reasonable assessment in our judgment. The battalion chaplain also dropped in on the sergeant's former section a couple times over the next month. The section performed well for the remainder of the operation. It appeared that although the sergeant was not forgotten, everyone was doing their job normally.

Centralized clinical services are necessary even when forward casualties are few. Nonbattle injuries can occur and precipitate crises requiring a prompt division mental health response. The CESD described here illustrates an unusually thorough debriefing process. The battalion commander was consulted first, and immediate steps were taken to meet with leaders as early as possible. The 91Gs were used to help ascertain the circle of crisis impact, including first witnesses and later medics, friends, and other unit members. Cooperation with chaplains in the debriefing and follow up process increased the immediacy of the intervention and the intensity of subsequent follow up. The debriefing itself involved convening the known witnesses, sharing of the witnessed events, and conducting a brief overview of useful soldier resources and common stress-related symptoms. The cooperation of command is always essential, and when the ordinance company commander objected to further mental health involvement, a request we felt obligated to comply with, the battalion chaplain became the more acceptable follow up alternative.

In retrospect, CESDs were ideally suited as a crisis intervention for the Gulf War. There were relatively few casualties, and the number of "hot spots" we needed to investigate was manageable. During periods of extended high-intensity combat, our ability to complete the steps outlined earlier might be sorely limited. Nevertheless, our experiences using CESDs suggest that their value in combat should not be underestimated, even when all steps cannot practically be completed.

CONCLUSIONS

In this chapter, we have reviewed a few of the many challenges the 1st Cavalry Division Mental Health Section faced during Operations Desert Shield and Desert Storm. The six C's of soldier, section, and mission Credibility, operational and logistical Cohesion, Combat stress prevention, Centralization of clinical services, forward deployed Contact teams, and Critical event stress debriefings were presented. We used them as our organizing principles during a very trying and often confusing overseas combat deployment. It is our hope that future division mental health teams might also find them helpful.

Some caveats to our approach merit mention. First, it has been suggested that during a high-intensity conflict the number of combat stress and battle fatigue casualties will quickly overwhelm DMHS resources and render small contact teams ineffectual. This may indeed be the case, but we would emphasize that contact teams may have the greatest utility in small operations or operations with relatively few casualties. Our emerging global military role seems to place us at greatest risk for participation in these kinds of skirmishes.

Second, breaking the section into four contact teams was a difficult decision that ultimately sacrificed some division mental health team operational cohesion to provide immediate and proximate assistance to maneuver elements. We later discovered that teams had experienced their own versions of the conflict and had generated their own unique identities and expectations founded on that experience. Working out our teams' divergent issues served as a laboratory for understanding the experiences of others when we returned home. For example, forward deployed contact teams returned to the rear of the division expecting that they had earned some rest and reward for their forward roles. Those on the rear team felt somewhat excluded from "the action" while simultaneously relieved they were safe. The rear team was anxious for the help of the forward teams, felt they had worked hard with relatively few accolades, and wanted appreciation from the forward team members. These differing perspectives resulted in transient section turmoil. Interestingly, analogous issues were at play when deployed units returned to Fort Hood. Returning soldiers felt much like members of the forward teams, while stateside soldiers saw things similarly to the rear contact team members. Overcoming these distinct perspectives was an ongoing reintegration process that took place both before and after our return to Fort Hood. While we later merged as a section and became a cohesive unit again, each team still identifies with their combat companies and brigades.

After returning to the states, we continued to rely on basic principles. We centralized garrison division mental health services by establishing the first all division mental health team clinic at Fort Hood since 1987. Our goal was to secure continued mental health advocacy for the division and maintain an avenue toward section cohesion and credibility. We continued to use contact teams, assigning one to each brigade as during the Gulf War.

One year after the ground conflict, the brigade involved in "busting the berm" went to the National Training Center (NTC). They specifically requested the same division mental health (contact) team they had during Desert Storm. During the exercise, a service was held for the brigade soldiers killed in Iraq. The mental health team members participated in the service.

ACKNOWLEDGMENT

The authors dedicate this chapter to the First Team soldiers killed in Operation Desert Storm. They live on in our memory and in the history of the 1st Cavalry Division.

REFERENCES

Bailey, P. (1918). "War neuroses, shell shock and nervousness in soldiers." *JAMA* 71: 2148–2153.

Braverman, M. (1992). "Posttrauma crisis intervention in the workplace." In J. C. Quick, L. R. Murphy, and J. J. Hurrell (eds.), *Stress & Well-Being at Work: Assessments and Interventions for Occupational Mental Health*. Washington, D.C.: American Psychological Association.

Engel, C. C. and S. J. Campbell. (in press). "Revitalizing division mental health in garrison: A post-Desert Storm perspective." *Mil. Med.*

Rahe, R. H. (1988). "Acute versus chronic psychological reactions to combat." *Mil. Med.*, 153:365–372.

Van Fleet, F. (1992). "Debriefing and the critical incident." *EAP Digest* 13:28–33.

8

Navy Combat Psychiatry in Support of Marine Forces in Ground Combat

Paul W. Ragan

INTRODUCTION

On December 1, 1990, I arrived at the 2nd Medical Battalion, 2nd Force Service Support Group (2nd FSSG), at Camp Lejeune, North Carolina, home of the II Marine Expeditionary Force (II MEF). Three weeks earlier, when President Bush had announced that he would deploy an additional 200,000 troops to Saudi Arabia, I was the head of the Outpatient Psychiatry Clinic at the National Naval Medical Center, Bethesda, Maryland. On November 27, 1990, just before I was scheduled to give a lecture to the residents on anxiety disorders, I was notified that I would deploy to the Gulf War as the psychiatrist for the 2nd Medical Battalion. I was selected, I was told, because I was a "Marine qualified" Navy psychiatrist, meaning I had previously been stationed at Camp Lejeune for three years. Fortunately, before I left Bethesda, I had the presence of mind to call the Department of Psychiatry at the Uniformed Services University of the Health Sciences (USUHS) and received a draft copy of the Army's Field Manual (FM–8–51) for Combat Stress Control in a Theater of Operations. I also received a message from a good psychologist friend of mine who was stationed with the Navy SEALS. He warned me that the medical doctrine supplied to the Marine Corps did not incorporate the basic principles of combat psychiatry and therefore did not mandate the mental health provisions necessary for treating a significant flow of combat stress casualties. In the 72 hours allotted to me to say good bye to my patients, my residents, and my family, there was no time to consider the implications of this assignment.

PHASE I: BRIDGING THE FIELD MEDICAL DOCTRINE GAP

The 2nd Medical Battalion was organized with a permanent staff, who provided the command structure and the administrative support staff augmented by Marines. During peacetime, a skeletal staff maintained the existence of the battalion. With the prospect of war, a Medical Personnel Unit Augmentation System (MPUAS) was activated and provided the battalion with its wartime table of organization, with medical personnel drawn from Navy medical commands scattered throughout the country.

On arrival, I inquired about the doctrine that governed the organization and operation of the battalion. I received a copy of the Fleet Marine Force Manual (FM) 4–50. Section 531–007 of this document noted that the treatment of wartime casualties required consideration of four interacting factors: the urgency and needs of the patient; the mobility and proximity of medical facilities to the operational forces; the medical capabilities of each echelon; and the volume of patient flow over a given period of time (i.e., the workload of each echelon of care).

It seemed a fairly simple matter of applying the expertise of combat psychiatry to these four factors. Unfortunately, what the manual dictated as the mental health capabilities of the 2nd Medical Battalion (a second echelon care facility) was a stress management team more appropriate to a *Fortune* 500 company than operational forces in a combat theater. The most forward elements of the battalion, the three collecting and clearing companies, were to have no mental health capabilities. The two surgical support companies were to have one psychologist each. The most rearward element, the headquarters and service company, was to have one psychiatrist, two psychologists, and four enlisted neuropsychiatric technicians. Together with the psychiatrist assigned to the division, that was the sum total of the mental health personnel assigned to the first two echelons of medical care (where the bulk of combat stress casualties must be treated) for an entire Marine Expeditionary Force totaling more than 40,000 personnel.

Shortly after arriving at Camp Lejeune, I was assigned to take an intensive version of the Medical Management of Chemical Casualties Course given by the U.S. Army. With the low cost of chemicals like Tabun, Sarin, and Soman, the ease of manufacture, and the rapid onset of toxic effects, it was no surprise that Iraqi President Saddam Hussein would consider their use. It soon became apparent to me that nerve agents were not as effective in killing large numbers of troops as they were in terrorizing them. The prospect of encountering these agents in the field had an extremely disquieting effect on the physicians taking the chemical casualties course and being briefed as to Hussein's variations on their use. One can imagine the effect on the rest of the military personnel being deployed to Southwest Asia.

One of the most valuable parts of FM–8–51 was Appendix B, "Predicting Combat Stress Workload." With the prospect of deploying in a few short weeks and not knowing when a ground war might commence, I found it useful to boil down the analysis for my superiors to three main factors: potential combat intensity (the United States was deploying over a half million troops to face who knows how many Iraqi troops in a geographical area about the size of the state of Iowa); the vast majority of our troops were "green" (i.e., without combat experience), whereas the majority of the Iraqi troops had combat experience from the war with Iran; and there was the high threat of chemical biological warfare.

We estimated that the contribution of psychiatric casualties to the patient flow volume would be on the average of one combat stress reaction (CSR) per three wounded-in-action (WIA). To increase the battalion's level of preparedness to handle such a volume of combat stress reactions, it was decided to divide the problem into four key elements—doctrine, command, personnel, and equipment—and tackle each one in turn. It is also suggested that the problems encountered locally in establishing the combat stress centers reflect similar problems at higher levels of the system. These four elements can serve as rubrics under which the successes and failures of the battalion as a whole can be categorized and better understood.

Doctrine

The first order of the day was to educate, even proselytize, to the command structure about the principles of combat psychiatry. My first entree was the executive officer of the battalion, who was able to recall a lecture on battle fatigue at his Command and Staff College given by an Air Force colonel. He was able to retrieve an article, interestingly enough, about German psychiatric casualties in World War II.

My first accomplishment was to deliver a point paper to the commanding officer of the battalion, which essentially was a short course on combat psychiatry, an estimate of the workload, and a proposal to create battalion level mental health units. As it turned out, this proposal was far too ambitious, and the required number of personnel was never provided. But it did provide a working doctrine with which the battalion could proceed.

Command Structure and Leadership Issues

The commander of the 2nd Medical Battalion was a health care administrator, and not a physician (he had previously served as a hospital comptroller). The executive officer was also a health care administrator as were the commanders of each of the medical companies. There were no physicians on the permanent battalion staff. There was a group surgeon on the staff of the Commanding General of the support group; he had no command authority and, regrettably, never made his presence felt throughout the entire campaign. The lack of medical leadership in the early stages of the battalion's deployment gave rise to numerous problems that extended far beyond the lack of planning for combat stress casualties.

One of the first inklings of the basic leadership problems was observed during the waning days before the first battalion party departed for overseas. Several junior enlisted members of the battalion's permanent staff who were followers of the Nation of Islam announced their refusal to deploy with the battalion. Supposedly, they were refusing to fight against fellow Muslims. This represented a serious breach of discipline. The manifest reason for their refusal appeared patently absurd, as a number of Islamic nations were contributing to the war effort against Iraq. Furthermore, a newly released book detailed a number of atrocities Hussein committed against the Muslim clergy in Iraq. I approached the acting sergeant major of the battalion with this observation and wondered what else was going on and was told in no uncertain terms to "butt out." The battalion leadership appeared uncertain about how to address the problem. The most outspoken of the young men was referred for psychiatric evaluation, which revealed no major psychopathology to account for the refusal to deploy. Rather than refer the men for charges and remove them from the battalion so they could no longer undermine morale, they were ordered to prepare for deployment despite their repeated refusals. Naturally, they became increasingly wedded to their defiant stance. In front of the families that had gathered to see the battalion commander and the advance party off, one of the young men refused to board the bus for the airfield. A fight broke out between him and a junior officer, and finally he was removed to the local brig and the advanced party departed.

Personnel

As noted previously, the medical battalion's wartime table of organization was filled by a system that consisted of requests to local hospital commanders for personnel representing specific specialties. However, the selection of whom to send was at the discretion of the local hospital commander. One of my first jobs was to direct the examination of individuals sent who appeared psychiatrically unfit or unsuitable for deployment. One would anticipate that assembling hundreds of people from dozens of commands to go to war would flush out individuals who were harboring psychological problems. Indeed, this occurred. For example, we saw one corpsman who had previously been on limited duty for depression, but then returned to full duty. With the stress of an anticipated deployment overseas, his minor depression recurred and he had to be referred for hospitalization.

From a group psychological point of view, we made two observations: Many people who were sent to join the battalion had just recently arrived at their parent commands. It appeared that the individuals to whom the parent commands were least attached were the ones selected for Persian Gulf duty. For example, my senior psychologist, on the day he checked into his new command at Twenty-nine Palms, was informed he was being deployed. Both his wife and his household goods were still in transit. Another health care professional, just married, was actually on his honeymoon when informed he had 24 hours to depart for Camp Lejeune. The other observation was that some commands appeared to use the call for personnel as a way of getting rid of "problem" individuals.

One individual came with a detailed neuropsychological assessment of his developmental learning disabilities. Another individual with an extensive history of poor performance reported to the medical battalion within three days of being discharged from his residency training program. This boded poorly for his success as a triage officer for a collecting and clearing company, which position he was to have filled. Not surprisingly, although he made it to Saudi Arabia before the depth of his problems was discovered, he had a stress reaction which required medical air evacuation back to the United States. The scramble to get this person out of country, send a message requesting a replacement, and pull someone to fill his position could have been avoided if his parent command had not sent him in the first place.

The commander of the battalion selected the chief of professional staff for the battalion based on seniority. Unfortunately, the individual selected did not work out. A new person was selected after the battalion arrived in Saudi Arabia. Unfortunately, this resulted in a loss of valuable time. Legitimate problems that arose went unresolved, conflict among the medical staff intensified, and the commander became increasingly impatient with what he perceived as medical staff bickering. For example, in reviewing their equipment needs, the orthopedic surgeons were divided on whether their tools should be air-or electricallypowered. Rather than recognizing that he or his chief of professional staff should take charge and direct problem solving and conflict resolution, the commander was observed to complain yet again about "those doctors."

PHASE II: WHAT WE FOUND UPON OUR ARRIVAL

Cognizant that we were part of the second half of the build-up, upon arrival in Al Jabail on December 24, 1990, I was very curious to see what personnel and organizational structure the 1st Medical Battalion, which had deployed earlier with I MEF, had put in place. I was particularly interested in what kind of preparations had been made for caring for combat stress casualties. I had heard that the Navy's surgeon general and the medical officer of the Marine Corps (coincidentally a psychiatrist) had preceded us by a week or two on a tour of the medical capabilities in the area. I expected to see something that would provide a model for my efforts.

What I found upon arrival shocked me. Astonishingly, the 1st Medical Battalion had deployed along with the rest of I MEF back in August without its commanding officer. In fact, he had arrived in country only about 10 days earlier and was scheduled for transfer in one to two months. As a consequence of this lack of leadership, the morale of the battalion and its mental health department were in shambles. This was reflected in an "epidemic" that broke out among the battalion medical personnel. The battalion chaplain estimated that about 30 of the professional staff found reason to return to the United States —most often on emergency leave, and most often never to return. This "epidemic" had totally disrupted the mental health department. The first psychiatrist that had deployed with the battalion had been so disagreeable that he was sent back to the United States after three weeks. The psychologist with Echo Company managed to return home on the strength of family problems. The Foxtrot Company psychologist reportedly eagerly deployed to the field; however, he ceased taking his ulcer medication. After he bled out twice, he too was sent back to the states. The remaining psychologist had recently secured emergency leave, and the current psychiatrist also departed for home on emergency leave, although the latter (to his credit) did return to Saudi Arabia when the crisis passed. The hoped-for months of advanced planning and preparation for combat stress casualties by the 1st Medical Battalion were not to be.

The situation at the first echelon of care (division psychiatrists) was also problematic. There was a psychiatrist in place with the 2nd Marine Division, which had deployed contemporaneously with us. However, the 1st Marine Division psychiatrist did not deploy with his division, and he had just arrived 10 days prior to us. Moreover, he sat out the entire first phase of the Gulf War in Al Jabail. When the division went through the breach of the mine fields on February 23, it was without its division psychiatrist. This situation was one of the symptoms, in this writer's opinion, of the powerlessness of medical authority and the lack of a hierarchical Marine medical command.

The situation was not much better with Fleet Hospital (FH 5), which represented the third echelon of care, or with its organic mental health team. FH 5 had been in place since September. By the time we arrived, dissatisfaction was rampant, and rumors abounded of women getting pregnant in order to be sent home, of congressional investigations, and of the imminent departure of the commanding officer.

FH 5's mental health department consisted of two psychiatrists, a senior psychologist, and a small number of psychiatric nurses and technicians staffing a 15 bed ward. The junior psychiatrist with whom I spoke exhibited chronic rage. He observed—as had others—that locating FH 5 on a tarmac in the middle of Al Jabail's industrial port needlessly exposed the hospital to attack. It was like "painting a target with the hospital as the bull's eye." Scud missile alerts were common. Besides its port, Al Jabail sat in the middle of an oil field, had an oil refinery, and sat at the north end of an industrial corridor which extended south to Ad Damman, Al Khubar, and Dhahran. Of the 72 Scud missiles the Iraqis fired, one of the last struck about 50 miles south of FH 5 at Dhahran and killed 28 Army soldiers.

Unfortunately, the mental health team at FH 5 chose to express their discontent by becoming a rogue element. This initially manifested itself by obstructionism when we sent them two patients requiring air evacuation back to the United States. Both were health care professionals determined to be unfit for duty. They were sent to us courtesy of abuses of the MPUAS system. One had been deployed without his antidepressant medication and had a serious recurrence of his mood disorder. The other was a medical officer who could not function in a medical residency program and had an extreme stress reaction when he mistook the burnt smell of an old window air conditioner for a gas attack. This patient was actually returned to 2nd Medical Battalion without prior notification. It took a conversation between commanding officers to get this situation rectified.

The relationship with the mental health team at FH 5 deteriorated further when we left Al Jabail and took up positions near the Kuwaiti border. After the air war had commenced, a corpsman in one of our medical companies made a serious suicide attempt. He took an overdose of Tylenol. There was a delay in finding him. He was unconscious and had no gag reflex. He required intubation and helicopter evacuation to FH 5. Afterward, I counted nine major risk factors for suicide in his history, including a prior attempt with a firearm, a family history of a completed suicide, and a history of an inheritable fatal disorder. Incredibly, he was returned to duty. His command was rather distressed and referred him to me. He was depressed, so I personally escorted him the 125 miles back to FH 5. Again, they returned him to his unit. Fortunately, a small airstrip was built next to our field hospital that could accommodate C 130s. I had the patient routed to a hospital in England. We had to maintain a suicide watch on him, however, for a week before his flight arrived.

When the ground war finally arrived, over 90 percent of the battle casualties were routed to FH 15 and not FH 5. Again, the conclusion appears inescapable that there was no medical chain of command that could effectively deal with dysfunctional elements as they became manifest.

Personnel

With the prospect of a high-intensity conflict and with the existing problems in preparedness at the first three echelons of care for battle fatigue, configuring combat stress centers was all the more paramount. The Army's combat stress control manual was an excellent blueprint, but the problem of personnel shortages had to be addressed. I had lost one psychologist, so we had three psychologists and four neuropsychiatric technicians. The immediate solution was to scale back from having mental health teams with each medical company. Discussions with the battalion commander revealed that the forward detachments were to be so lightweight and mobile that they could not support the treatment and return to duty of combat stress casualties.   Therefore, I decided that with such limited personnel it would be best to construct 45 bed combat stress centers, one at each surgical support company. My colleagues hit on the solution to scour the battalion for suitable general-duty corpsmen. In this way, an additional 10 corpsmen were selected and trained to function as psychiatric technicians. Certainly, we had to have the battalion commander's support to do this. The main problem with recruiting corpsmen this way was that they had to "come out of hide," which meant they were taken out of their respective companies (this did not endear us to their company commanders). Therefore, two mental health professionals and seven corpsmen were to staff each center until additional personnel arrived.

Since the bias of the medical doctrine in FM–4–50 was to make field hospitals surgically intensive, one obvious solution was to request the deployment of additional mental health professionals. To this end, I pushed for a meeting with the senior medical officer in the region. With my counterpart from 1st Medical Battalion and others, I met the senior Marine surgeon on December 29, 1990 to outline the anticipated volume of combat stress casualties, the need for CSCs, and the personnel to staff them. In due course, the senior surgeon agreed to send the request to the United States. Several days later, I was called to the camp commandant's office to receive a telephone call from the surgeon. He was calling to say he had sent the message requesting the additional mental health personnel. However, the real purpose of his call appeared to be some good natured grousing. He had thought just prior to sending the message to call stateside to brief the senior medical officer of the Marine Corps, who (as was noted earlier) happened to be a psychiatrist. He wondered what his opinion of our request was, and he thought to give him advance notice before the message arrived. However, the surgeon was informed that the medical officer of the Marine Corps was on annual leave out of state to see one of the New Year's college bowl games and could not take his call. This was two weeks before the air war phase of the Gulf War was scheduled to start.

Equipment

If the wartime table of organization for mental health professionals within the battalion was deficient, at least it existed. The problem of the wartime table of equipment (T/E) can be stated more simply: It did not exist. Basically, we had to invent everything needed to create a 45 bed combat stress-control center. This included making sure the center was included in the camp plans and not located next to Graves Registration, but close to the showers. More than once the center was "omitted" from the camp plans. Then, starting with the T/E for a basic medical ward of a collecting and clearing company, we added everything needed to make it a functional center.   This included additional chemical protective suits for stress casualties expected to arrive without theirs; restraint sets, syringes, needles, Haloperidol, Benztropine, and Diphenhydramine for psychotic cases; and Chlorpromazine, Diazepam, Flurazepam, and Lorazepam for less severe cases or as one time sleepers. Medical documentation forms were designed and printed on the units' administrative computer For the next war, considering all the contingencies, a complete, self contained psychiatric/combat stress AMAL (Authorized Medical II Allowance List) needs to be designed, prepared, and placed with the battalion assets.

There was one piece of equipment which was too big for me to get my hands on, but which experts in the field recognize as indispensable for the combat psychiatrist: a vehicle. Considering that I was tasked with delivering stress lectures to forward logistics groups, attending medical group meetings back at Al Jabail, and visiting battalion assets and trouble spots scattered from the outskirts of Kuwait City to Al Jaber Airport to our combat stress centers at Al Khanjar and Abraq Al Kibrit in the desert to Al Mishab, a vehicle would have saved me an enormous amount of time spent hitch-hiking.

PHASE III: DEPLOYING COMBAT STRESS CENTERS IN THE DESERT

The last obstacle to deploying a field hospital and its attendant combat stress centers to the desert came from an unexpected source. Al Kibrit was selected as the initial site for the direct support command and the two surgical support companies with their combat stress centers. This site was 25 miles due west of Al Mishab and 30 miles south of the Al Wafrah oil fields. Little did we know at the time that this was as far north and west as military planners wanted us to be prior to Iraqi surveillance capabilities being knocked out. Twenty year old decommissioned city buses were allocated to transport Foxtrot Company from Al Jabail to Al Kibrit. The elements of nature then transpired. On January 12, 1991, the rain began. We left in the early afternoon on January 13. Most of the company became mired in the mud on the stretch from Al Mishab to Al Kibrit. Nine hours later, two trucks and one bus managed to struggle into camp. The rest of the company spent the night stuck until they could be retrieved the following day.

Once actually in the field, life took a different turn. The focus became to set up the hospital and the combat stress center. This was somewhat therapeutic. On January 20, 1991, the hospital officially opened for business and we saw our first stress casualty (mild) brought on mainly by having been deployed without his corrective lenses and being assigned to nighttime "lock and load" (weapons loaded and ready to fire) searches in the desert. Forty-two of the 50 odd cases seen at the two combat stress centers at Al Kibrit were returned to their units. My senior psychologist was especially effective at treating a number of "gas mask phobia" cases referred to us.

Two related problems deserve at least brief mention because of their potential magnitude to disrupt and/or halt field hospital operations. The first is that no provisions were made for proper decontamination of chemically exposed casualties. Fortunately for the battalion, we had a pediatrician with a Ph.D. in toxicology who designed and built from scratch decontamination equipment, the components of which he literally had "to beg, borrow, and steal." Since this equipment was untried, he remained doubtful to the end how well we could have handled even a small load of contaminated casualties.

The other problem concerned the nerve agent pretreatment strategy. What are the psychopharmacological implications of treating masses of troops with 30 milligrams every eight hours of pyridostigmine bromide? Sitting in the field taking my pyridostigmine tablets, three issues presented themselves: How many cases of subclinical asthma or dysrhythmia would be uncovered by this medication? What impact would the side effect profile (especially GI symptoms in a desert environment) have on compliance? Are there cognitive impairments induced by this combination, possibly additive from both increased cholinergic activity and bromide intoxication? We attempted to investigate the latter by field cognitive testing on the day of and seven days into taking the medication. This project had to be abandoned when we discovered compliance was so poor because of side effects.

CONCLUSION

This chapter has highlighted a number of significant problems encountered in the process of organizing, preparing, deploying, and operating a credible combat mental health system in support of Marine and Navy combat operations during the Gulf War. Detailed information was provided related to specific issues like combat mental health doctrine, command structure and leadership issues, personnel and equipment, and actual deployment experiences in the initial staging areas as well as in a forward deployed position. The author hopes that these details will provide concrete lessons for those who will have the responsibility to carry out future combat deployments. While some of these issues and some of the author's experiences are unique to the nature of the Gulf War, the lessons here will no doubt prove valuable in the range of conflicts that are surely to occur in the future.

Part II

COPING WITH THE EXPERIENCE OF COMBAT

9

After-Action Critical Incident Stress Debriefings and Battle Reconstructions Following Combat

Gregory Belenky, James A. Martin, and Scott C. Marcy

INTRODUCTION

This chapter describes the use of after action critical incident stress debriefing and battle reconstruction techniques as mental health interventions with combat arms soldiers immediately following battlefield engagements. The authors served with the U.S. Army 2nd Armored Cavalry Regiment (2 ACR) during the Persian Gulf War. The first two authors were members of a five-person mental health team attached to the medical troop of the regimental support squadron. The third author was a squadron commander. The 2 ACR led the U.S. Army VIIth Corps sweep around the Iraqi left flank through Iraq and into Kuwait. The mission of the 2 ACR was to find and to fix in place the Iraqi Republican Guards for subsequent destruction by the U.S. Army 1st and 3rd Armored Divisions. These divisions followed the 2 ACR into Iraq.

The 2 ACR accomplished its mission. The 2 ACR also experienced death and injury of unit members, which are the inevitable consequences of war.

BACKGROUND

At the time of the Gulf War, The 2 ACR was a smaller than division-sized unit usually composed of approximately 6500 soldiers. It included four combat squadrons (battalion sized units); three composed of armor (M1 tanks) and mechanized infantry scouts (Bradley fighting vehicles) and one composed of attack helicopters. In addition, there was a regimental support squadron, which includes a medical troop. For the Gulf War, the 2 ACR was augmented by other units, including an artillery brigade, transportation units, explosive ordnance disposal personnel, and additional medical support, including a mental health team. As configured during the Gulf War, the 2 ACR's strength was 9500 soldiers, a base of 6500 plus an additional 3000.

Prior to the Gulf War, mental health personnel in the Army were, by doctrine, deployed at the division level. Thus the 2 ACR deployed to the Gulf region from its home station in Germany with no mental health personnel in its medical troop. The regimental surgeon, appreciating that with its many attachments the 2 ACR was approaching the size of a small division, requested mental health support from VIIth Corps. A mental health team was formed, consisting of two psychiatrists, a social worker, and a behavioral science specialist. The team joined the 2 ACR on February 10, 1991, fourteen days before the beginning of the ground war.

From past experience of the American and other armies, we expected both acute and chronic stress casualties to emerge in those elements engaged in combat, in those in which friendly fire incidents occurred, and in those in which there were deaths or injuries from other causes (e.g., vehicular accidents, unexploded ordnance, etc.). To treat acute stress casualties, we planned brief forward treatment, consisting of rest, sleep, physical replenishment (water and food), and a chance for stress casualties to tell their story to a comprehending and sympathetic person, followed by the soldier's rapid return to duty with his or her own unit. Whenever possible, we planned to conduct this treatment in situ without removing the stress casualty from his or her unit and comrades. Whenever possible, we planned to combine treatment of the acute casualty with a more general, less clinical, postcombat debriefing and battle reconstruction for other members of the soldier's immediate unit. To foster unit reintegration, to gain operational lessons for future combat, and to reduce the risk of subsequent posttraumatic stress disorder (PTSD), we planned to do postcombat debriefings with all units in the 2 ACR that were involved in combat during the ground war.

BEFORE THE GROUND WAR

The mental health team spent the 14 days prior to the beginning of the ground war introducing themselves to the soldiers of the 2 ACR. We would go to a unit and walk the screen line, from M1 tank to M1 tank, from Bradley fighting vehicle to Bradley fighting vehicle, introducing ourselves as part of the mental health team of the 2 ACR. We explained that we would be available during the ground war if anyone encountered difficulty, and that we would be back after the cease-fire to reconstruct with them the events of the ground war. We were received warmly and with interest, and we were impressed that the farther forward we went, the more relaxed and confident soldiers were.

In the scouts who were to be the most forward element in the advance, we were hard put to find even mild cases of butterflies in anticipation of the coming ground offensive. This was, we believe, for a variety of reasons. The morale and cohesion of the combat elements were high. The majority of soldiers had known each other and trained together for the past two years. The soldiers had confidence in the technical superiority of their equipment. They knew that they could see (with thermal imaging sight) and hit (with antitank missiles and kinetic energy rounds) the Iraqis before the Iraqis could see or hit them. Finally, they were receiving current intelligence on the accelerating destruction of Iraqi armored and mechanized infantry by Coalition air strikes.

COMBAT

The beginning of the ground war (G Day) was February 24, 1991. Combat operations by 2 ACR began a day earlier on February 23 at 1310 hours. At 1330, the 210th Field Artillery Brigade, attached as artillery support to the 2 ACR, opened with a barrage of howitzer and Multiple Launch Rocket System (MLRS) fire on suspected Iraqi positions. Immediately following the barrage, the 2nd and 3rd Squadrons of the 2 ACR advanced into Iraq, reaching their objective by 1530 without contact with the enemy. Intelligence suggested that on G Day, as the 2 ACR continued its advance into Iraq, it would encounter scattered disorganized infantry, on G+1 (February 25) better organized mechanized infantry, and on G+2 (February 26) well-organized armor in the form of the Iraqi Republican Guards. This is substantially what happened. On G Day (February 24) and G+1 (February 25), the 2 ACR advanced initially north, then northeast, picking up surrendering Iraqi infantry and mechanized infantry soldiers. Early on G+2 (February 26), the 2 ACR turned due East and met and engaged the Republican Guards. Fighting continued until late in the evening. Late on G+2, the following 1st and 3rd Armored Divisions began passing through and around the 2 ACR and took over the battle. At 0200 hours on G+3 (February 27), the 2 ACR ceased fire and became the VIIth Corps reserve force. A general cease-fire went into effect at 0800 on G+4 (February 28), ending the ground war. After the cease-fire, the 2 ACR proceeded east into Kuwait, arriving in its designated area on March 1, 1991.

We began our debriefings on March 3, conducting them in the same systematic fashion as we had made our introductions prior to the ground war. We went to the combat elements and proceeded from tank to tank, from fighting vehicle to fighting vehicle, reconstructing day by day and, as appropriate, minute by minute the events of the ground war. We typically began the process with a discussion about crossing the berm into Iraq and finished with the arrival of the unit in Kuwait. We interviewed each crew separately. We used information gathered from previous crews to shed light on the situation of the crew we were debriefing at the moment. All the personnel we interviewed were interested and eager to tell their story. Often, we were told that we were the first people to come to talk to them to find out what had happened. Next we describe three of the debriefings to illustrate the technique and demonstrate its value.

CASUALTIES AND THE DEBRIEFING PROCESS

Case 1: An Accidental Death

On the evening of February 28 (the cease-fire had gone into effect at 0800 hours that morning), as the 2 ACR was moving into Kuwait, a headquarters troop was establishing camp for the night. They had moved their vehicles into a coil, which means a circular defensive arrangement with tanks and fighting vehicles facing outward. The men were digging foxholes in front of their vehicles. One young soldier, a member of a fighting vehicle crew, was digging his foxhole when his vehicle commander called him back to his vehicle. The soldier turned, shouldered his shovel, and accidentally stepped on an unexploded American Dual Purpose Improved Conventional Munitions (DPICM), covered by sand, which exploded. The soldier was carrying rifle grenades in an ammunition vest on his chest. These exploded as well. The soldier was in all probability killed outright.

Two medics, both young and inexperienced (just out of school) enlisted soldiers, who had completed their training only a few months before joining the 2 ACR and had joined this particular troop only a few weeks before, tried to resuscitate the soldier. The resuscitation was gruesome. As they tried to ventilate the soldier, air escaped from his cheek, so someone put a hand there. Then air escaped from the chest, so someone put a hand there. Then air escaped from the abdomen, so someone put a hand there. Finally, air escaped from one eye socket. The medics continued their efforts for about 20 minutes, at which point a physician from the medical troop arrived, assessed the situation as hopeless, and called off the resuscitation.

Two days later, we were asked to see one of the medics because he was clearly distressed by what had happened. We responded that we would see him. We also commented to the unit leader that if this soldier was so obviously distressed, this probably indicated less obvious but still significant distress in others who had been involved in the resuscitation, in the soldier's comrades, and in his immediate chain of command. We proposed therefore to assemble all involved, including the two medics, the others involved in the resuscitation, the soldier's comrades, and the immediate chain of command and do a debriefing and reconstruction of the accident and resuscitation and relevant events before and after. The unit leader agreed to our proposal.

We assembled the group in the open air and arranged cots in a circle for everyone to sit on. We began the debriefing by suggesting that for the purpose of reconstructing events, rank be set aside and that all participants be accorded the status of equal witnesses. The debriefing took 2.5 hours. In the course of the debriefing, the events of the resuscitation, as outlined earlier in this chapter, were presented in vivid detail. The medic whom we had been asked to see twice got up and stood in the center of the group, and with his eyes focused on infinity described what he had seen and done during the resuscitation. The other medic contributed.

The soldier's vehicle commander described the events surrounding the soldier's stepping on the unexploded bomblet. The soldier's friends initially expressed reservations about the competency of the medics and whether all that could and should have been done to try and save their friend was done. It was in response to these expressed misgivings that the more affected medic stood in the center of the group and described the resuscitation. During his vivid and detailed recounting, it became obvious to those friends of the soldier who had not been present at the time of the accident that the two medics had done the best they could and that they had done more than the soldier's friends could easily imagine themselves doing. As he spoke, the medic visibly became less distressed and equally visibly gained confidence and self assurance. Concerns over the quality of the resuscitation in the soldier's friends quickly receded.

The soldier's immediate chain of command raised another issue. Just before the ground war, the soldier's wife had given birth. The mother and child were fine, but by U.S. Army regulation the soldier met the requirements to be granted emergency leave to go home to visit his wife and child. The chain of command and the soldier discussed this and mutually agreed that since there was no problem at home, the soldier should stay with the unit and go through the ground war with his comrades, and then go home. This decision was reexamined by the group in the light of subsequent events. In retrospect, everyone wished the soldier had gone home. However, the group consensus was that the decision was the correct one at the time, and that faced with similar circumstances in the future, the decision would likely be the same.

The soldier's friends raised another issue. The soldier, at the time he stepped on the bomblet, was carrying several rifle grenades, and these in turn exploded, contributing further to his injuries. The fact that he was carrying these grenades at all had been a concern to some of his friends and to his chain of command. The soldier had no compelling reason to be carrying them once the cease-fire went into effect. He apparently felt more confident with them and was reluctant to give them up. It was clear that no one pushed the soldier to give up his grenades out of respect for his feelings about the matter. In retrospect, both comrades and chain of command wished they had taken a firmer stance with respect to the grenades.

By the end of the debriefing, everyone had a clearer view of the accident, its antecedents, and the resuscitation. For the medic who was most affected, it was clearly a turning point both in terms of how he viewed himself and in how his comrades viewed him. By the end of the debriefing, the medic was clearly free of distress, and his comrades viewed him with a new respect. From that point, he became a valued, well-thought-of member of the unit, whereas before, from our own observations of him, he had been treated with little regard and was clearly on the periphery of things.   On follow-up, several weeks later, he continued to do very well.

Case 2: Death by Friendly Fire

As we proceeded with our systematic debriefings of combat elements, we debriefed units in the 2 ACR involved in two related instances of friendly fire. On G+1 (February 25), combat elements of the 2 ACR were advancing over open desert.   They consisted of platoons of six Bradley infantry fighting vehicles, each platoon supported by a platoon of four M1 tanks. The formation was a line of Bradleys followed a kilometer or two behind by a line of M1s. As the elements advanced, their principal activity was taking the surrender of disorganized Iraqi infantry. One platoon of Bradleys was accompanied by two older, less well protected M113 armored personnel carriers, whose task was to look after the approximately 80 Iraqi prisoners that the unit had captured. At circa 1800 hours, the advance was halted for the day. The Bradleys deployed in a screen line facing east, the M1s deployed a kilometer or two to their rear, and the M113s with their Iraqi prisoners took a position 50 to 100 meters in front of the Bradleys' screen line.

At 0205 hours on G+2 (February 26), six Iraqi armored personnel carriers, apparently elements of an Iraqi mechanized infantry battalion, were observed advancing northwest toward the screen line.   The Iraqis were in column formation. Because of rain and wind blown sand, visibility even with thermal imaging sights was poor. The lead Iraqi vehicle was actually in the screen line in the vicinity of the Bradleys on the platoon's left flank before either side understood that they were encountering the enemy.

Several things happened at once. A firefight erupted, involving the Bradleys of the platoon itself, the Bradleys of the flanking platoon on the left, and, after an interval, the supporting M1s. The two M113s securing the Iraqi prisoners requested and received permission to withdraw toward the rear. The Iraqi prisoners themselves began running in panic in all directions, some of them climbing onto the American vehicles for safety. The Iraqi vehicles were quickly destroyed.

The two Bradleys on the left flank of the platoon were maneuvering in and around the burning Iraqi vehicles. They were mistaken for Iraqis by the Bradleys constituting the platoon's right flank, who fired on them with their 25-millimeter cannons. Both Bradleys on the left were destroyed. Fortunately, as a result of the crew safety provisions of the Bradleys (Halon fire suppression, Kevlar spall curtain, etc.), both crews of five escaped unhurt and were picked up still unscathed by their comrades.

The crews of the withdrawing M113s were not so fortunate. As they withdrew to the rear, they became misoriented, and instead of proceeding directly rearward, they veered off toward the left flank of the platoon, crossing over into the gap between the platoon of Bradleys on the left and their supporting M1s. The M1s at the beginning of the firefight were some distance to the rear and were rapidly moving forward to support their Bradleys. They knew nothing about the presence of the M113s. They observed the M113s proceeding in front of, and collinear with, the column of burning Iraqi vehicles and, taking them to be Iraqis, destroyed them both.

The drivers of both M113 vehicles were killed outright. The survivors dismounted their vehicles, only to be pursued once on the ground by the M1s. During this pursuit, which included one M1 coming around a second time and firing on them with its coaxial machine gun, three more soldiers were killed outright or so severely wounded that they died before first light. The remaining soldiers, wounded and unwounded, were picked up at first light. Out of a total of 12 crew members in both M113s, five were killed, six were wounded, and only one came through uninjured. This one uninjured soldier went on to develop a clear case of posttraumatic stress disorder, which is the third case we will discuss later in this chapter.

We debriefed all the unevacuated personnel involved in these friendly fire incidents, including the crews of both the principal and the flanking platoon of Bradleys, and the crews of the M1s. The account which we have given of the events is based on these debriefings. With all the crews, we began with the beginning of the ground war and the crossing of the berm on February 24th. This was despite considerable pressure from the crews themselves to begin immediately with the friendly fire incidents. We explained that the full reconstruction was necessary in order for us and them to be able to place events in their proper context.

The story as we have described it was not known in full by any one person when we began our debriefings. By the end of the debriefing, a clear and shared picture had emerged. The crews we debriefed were appreciative of the opportunity to tell their story. They related that before the ground war, all echelons of higher command had come to visit them and give them encouragement. Since the cease-fire, we were, in their view, the first to show any interest. This was despite the fact that the squadron commander (the third author) had been visiting each of his units every day and that the U.S. Army historical team had been through just ahead of us, as had the officer investigating the friendly fire incidents.

In friendly fire incidents, denial, anger, and guilt are common among those involved. Often, these incidents are not looked at closely for fear of focusing responsibility on a few people, who then would be receptacles for all that was bad in the unit. We found that the effect of our debriefings and reconstructions was quite the opposite. Although our reconstructions made clear who in fact had put the cross hairs on the target and pulled the trigger, they also made abundantly clear that it was a series of mistakes and misjudgments by many people that made the friendly fire incident possible. Others perceived that they were not without responsibility. They might also have pulled the trigger under similar circumstances. Thus, as the facts became clearer as a result of the reconstruction of events, the actual responsibility was more accurately distributed and, at least in the present instances, reduced scapegoating and blame. Finally, valuable operational lessons were learned about how to prevent such instances in the future.

Case 3: Addressing Posttraumatic Stress

In the crews of the M113s destroyed by friendly fire in the early hours of G+2 (February 26), there was one soldier out of the twelve who came through uninjured. This soldier had attempted to give first aid to the wounded and had made repeated attempts to get help, including going back to the vehicle and trying to use the radio and finally at first light sending up flares. The flares and improving visibility finally brought help. The soldier later developed acute posttraumatic stress disorder (PTSD). He had intrusive thoughts of the event while awake, he had nightmares and vivid dreams of the event, and he became anxious, fearful, withdrawn, and ineffective. He wanted nothing to do with armored vehicles of any sort. Due to his symptoms, he was reassigned to the 2 ACR's rear detachment located in Northern Saudi Arabia. He continued to do poorly after this reassignment.

The first author, a psychiatrist, was visiting the rear detachment and was asked to see the soldier. It would have been preferable to see the soldier in situ in his unit and to do the debriefing and reconstruction in a group including his friends and comrades and his immediate chain of command. As his unit was with the main body of the 2 ACR in Iraq, this was not possible. Fortunately, we had already conducted the debriefing and reconstruction with the other personnel involved, as described earlier. So the first author knew the story in detail. He met with the soldier and included in the meeting both a close friend of the soldier who was also assigned to the rear detachment and the rear detachment commander. Assembling this group, the author spent two hours going over the events of the ground war from the soldier's perspective.

The soldier described in vivid detail the destruction of the M113 and the wounding and deaths of his comrades. He described one of the wounded men, clearly dying, praying out loud that the M1 tank which had destroyed their M113 and had then systematically hunted them down on the ground would not return. He described his repeated trips to the destroyed M113 to try to raise help on the radio and to get additional supplies. He described his finally successful attempt to get help using flares. The soldier was tearful and agitated at many points in the reconstruction. By the end, he was calmer. Subsequently, his symptoms subsided and he was able to return to duty with his unit in Iraq. Once back with his unit, his squadron commander (the third author) spent some time with him reviewing the experience and supporting him. He continued to do well.

The squadron commander (third author) conducted troop (company)-level after-action debriefings and battle reconstructions after the 2 ACR had returned to its home base in Germany. Again, the effect was to distribute responsibility for the things that had gone wrong. It became clear that when things went right, this was the result not of one person making a correct decision, but rather of a series of people making correct decisions. The process served to share both blame and credit.

SUMMARY

Prevention of combat stress casualties depends on morale, leadership, cohesion, training, fitness, and a variety of other personal and unit factors. Battle intensity and battle type are also important determinants of the incidence of combat stress casualties. Acute combat stress casualties are best treated forward with a brief rest, physical replenishment (water, food, and sleep), and a chance to tell one's story followed by a rapid return to duty with one's own unit.

There were no acute stress casualties in the 2 ACR during the 100 hours of the ground war. What physical casualties there were primarily resulted from accident or incidents of friendly fire. Our mental health efforts therefore focused on after action debriefings and battle reconstructions. We used this as a general, prophylactic intervention for all soldiers who had seen action, as a specific intervention in cases of accident or friendly fire, and as a form of individual intervention, though conducted in a group, for anyone identified as a stress casualty. We found this to be an effective technique in all instances. Through consultation, we encouraged others (small unit leaders, chaplains, and other medical personnel) to use this intervention technique.

In our own debriefings, we were frequently assisted by physicians from the medical troop. After action debriefings provided accurate information to the participants regarding the true nature of the events. Responsibility became both clear and more generally shared. For distressed individuals and identified stress casualties, the technique provided symptomatic relief, fostered reintegration into the unit and return to effective duty, improved well-being, and promoted personal growth. For the unit, the technique restored morale and cohesion and provided valuable operational lessons for the future. We believe that the work of military mental health personnel does not end with the end of the battle and that after action debriefings and battle reconstructions by both mental health personnel and commanders should be standard practice in combat units.

10

Mental Health Interventions for the Survivors of a Scud Missile Attack

Joyce C. Humphrey

INTRODUCTION

We were at war now, a ground war. The sky was clear; only the desert can create such a clear sunset and night skyline as it contrasts with the flat surface. The air was still. On this fateful night, as I reached the mess hall, this sense of peace was quickly destroyed. Alarms went off, shattering the silence: first the alarms from the King Abul Aziz Air Base, and then the distant alarms from the surrounding towns. The alarms continued as the sky suddenly filled with a fresh brilliance. Was this an incoming Scud? So close?

We all ran for cover and donned our masks. All was confusion inside the mess hall: Some had their gas masks on, some were calmly eating their meals, and some were running around without apparent purpose. A young sergeant came into the mess hall and reported to the General, who was present at dinner, that a Scud had hit. He was very calm. He made it seem like this happened every day. He did not seem alarmed and did not mention where the Scud had hit.

The alarms ended. It was time to return to headquarters. There was no sense of urgency. The sky was again clear. The air was calm. There was no hint of the tragedy that had just occurred.

As I arrived at my post in the headquarters building, I was almost knocked over by an ambulance team running to their vehicle "to reach the victims of the Scud attack!" The confusion, noise, multiple conversations utilizing every form of communication available, and the sudden barrage of questions confirmed my worst fears—a Scud had hit an American compound. Would there be more? The air and ground ambulances had already been dispatched along with a trauma team from one of the Army hospitals. It sounded like things were under control.

A CALL FOR HELP

A request came in to send a team to assist with the victims of the Scud attack, estimated to be approximately 160 soldiers. The exact number was unknown. Those who were not seriously injured were enroute to a safe location, a large steel structure called the EXPO. Approximately half the size of a football field, it had already been filled with a few hundred beds, some privacy curtains, outside showers, a first aid station, and a refreshments table. The building was normally used to receive incoming military replacements from the United States.

Around midnight, the alarms sounded again but this time it sounded on deaf ears. The soldiers from the Scud attack were arriving via buses and being offloaded just as the alarms sounded. Their gait was slow. All facial expression was gone; cuts and facial abrasions were evident. Their uniforms were torn and often blood stained. Their weapons, gas masks, jackets, and in some cases even their boots were missing. Their eyes seemed to stare over your head, and they did not seem to hear what you were saying. They slowly straggled into the building; each soldier took a moment to look up at the ceiling filled with large steel beams and flood lights. The ceiling seemed to pose a greater threat than the alarms. Unseen pieces of fiberglass from the explosion were soon everywhere, causing most to itch.

As the soldiers realized their physical discomfort, they proceeded through the showers, donned new clothing, used the latrines, and sought some refreshment. Some chose to sit on the beds and stare into space. Small groups of two or three soldiers began to cluster together. One soldier proudly paraded in with the unit guidon torn and stained but still attached to the pole. He tied the pole to his new bed, gathering his friends to his side. As the group settled in, the quiet gloom was soon replaced by a steady noise as the soldiers retold their stories to each other, as if for the first time.

RESPONDING TO ACUTE PSYCHOLOGICAL STRESS

Our plan was to act as catalysts and encourage those who wanted to talk to do so; those that only wanted to sit and have a companion were given the space. Our team consisted of eight chaplains, one psychiatrist, and one nurse. Those with minor injuries were sent to the first aid station; some of the soldiers in their haste to help their fallen companions had ignored ear, eye, and other facial injuries. Each of the team members circulated between the beds, sitting with the small groups for a period of time and then moving on quietly to a new group or an individual.

Each soldier was eventually seen by one of the team. Some wanted to tell their story; some just wanted to sit and cry. One sergeant had just been assigned her platoon and had now lost all of them; she said, "What do I do now?" She had lost her flashlight and could not remember where or when. She felt lost and alone. Another female soldier stayed with her for the remainder of the night.

The phones that might be able to get a message north were all down, and a portion of the unit located on the Iraq boarder still did not know that the rest of the unit had been hit. The officer in charge of getting this message north felt compelled to call over and over in a vain attempt to reach their forward detachment; one of their chaplains was at the border. The soldier commented, "I would want to know if it happened to my people." Eight hours of trying to call were finally rewarded at 0800. The soldier had not showered or taken care of any personal needs; his only objective had been to notify the unit members in the north.

SUFFERING AMONG THE SURVIVORS

Cries of anguish and despair were repeatedly heard. One soldier after another stated, "I could not do enough." "I knew what to do, I remembered my ABC's in the manual but I did not have enough bandages or splints." "They were dying and I could not get them all out." The flames, the noise, the confusion, the explosions, "like bullets," were all terrifying. "There were cars everywhere, lights flashing, people—Arab and American. I did not know if we were under attack or if all those people were there to help." "They were my buddies, I've lost _____." One young male soldier, crying, blood on his hands, staring into space, said, "I never saw part of a person before, a girl, her arm was off, can you imagine it? She's dead, my God, she's dead. I could not find the arm, someone wanted the arm. I'd never seen people hurt before, so many body parts unattached. I felt helpless."

A female soldier said, "I felt part of a team here [in Saudi] much more than at home. We were together to do something important." When asked what she had been able to give to her fallen soldiers, she said, "Only caring, love, a move to safety, check their wounds, not much, not enough, too many died as I watched, as I tried to hold on and shout hold on, don't go. It wasn't enough and it could have been me. Why not me?"

Some of the soldiers found it impossible to sleep inside the EXPO. All they could see were the large steel beams overhead, and they had seen the same picture in the now destroyed warehouse just up the road. They slept in the buses. Some soldiers could not cry. Many kept commenting on the blood, the open stomachs, the cut-off arms or legs. One soldier commented, "I never saw that stuff before and I hope I never do again. I could only move them out. I could not stop all the bleeding and loss of arms and legs. Remember that girl with her arm missing? God, it was awful. I think I knew her."

For most of the survivors, the scene was confusing, frightening, and overwhelming. They had difficulty making any sense out of what had happened and in their own role after the Scud hit. Most could not recall where they had spent the three hours prior to their arrival at EXPO. Almost every one commented, "All I could do was get them out of the building; I had to get them out." Not one soldier had expressed any concern for his or her own safety after the missile hit. Very few had put on masks, gathered weapons, or sought personal protection. All had headed directly for the warehouse to "save their buddies, to pull them out."

A THERAPEUTIC MISTAKE

Our plan was effective. The soldiers' basic needs were being met. Each was given a safe environment (if any place is safe in a war zone), food, a shower, and clean clothes. New protective masks and gear would have to wait until morning. This group had survived, but not without paying a painful price. Each soldier would need more time and more help. Due to the availability of overseas commercial telephone lines, many of these soldiers had called home from the EXPO, relieving their own families but, unknown to them, only increasing the anxiety of the families that did not hear from their soldiers. One young man had been talking to his father when the Scud hit. His last words to his father had been, "Oh, my God,___," and the line went dead. He was one of the first to call home.

The next day, a mental health team from an area Army hospital was assigned to assist the soldiers in the survival group. This team of four arrived at EXPO around 0500 and remained with the soldiers for the next 48 hours. This team attempted to group the survivors by their own intervention criteria (i.e., age, sex, or rank) rather than leaving soldiers in their normal unit groupings. The soldiers resisted these efforts and later reported this period to be nonproductive. The soldiers felt this intervention was not helpful. Some soldiers expressed resentment that these outsiders were there telling them what to do. They did not want to talk about the attack anymore. They did not want to talk to strangers; they did not need help.

THE DAYS THAT FOLLOWED

After two days, most of the soldiers were moved back into their original barracks, which were still standing adjacent to the destroyed warehouse. For some, the building's remains became a monument to the fallen soldiers, a very private area. Some of the soldiers left within 24 hours to drive their much-needed supplies forward; the troops would be relying on the fuel, water, and food their trucks would deliver. The unit's mission was never interrupted (a fact of true pride frequently mentioned by these soldiers).

Within 24 hours, the 28 dead were accounted for, prepared for flight, and flown to Dover, Delaware. All the personal belongings of the dead, injured, and survivors in the warehouse were gathered and painstakingly inventoried by the unit's assigned staff. Within seven days, the majority of wounded had been airevacuated to U.S. medical facilities in Europe (56) and America (18). The last Scud victim remained in Bahrain, too critical to survive a flight until April 1. The survivors (26 slightly injured and 100 other unit members) remained in Saudi Arabia, performing their mission, until May 15, when they redeployed back to the United States.

The injured all processed through local U.S. military hospitals in Saudi Arabia prior to either being returned to duty or evacuated out of the combat theater of operations. Each of these hospitals had only one psychiatrist and one psychiatric nurse. Each of these individuals had a primary war assignment in an acute patient care role. The priority was placed on the physical injuries, preparing patients for evacuation, and meeting the theater's seven-day evacuation policy. Under these conditions, it was nearly impossible to attend to mental health issues, a fact of frustration to the patient and the mental health staff. The 74 soldiers from the Scud attack, who were evacuated from Saudi within three to four days, received minimal, if any, mental health intervention.

The unit chaplains remained in touch with these soldiers on a daily basis, keeping track of those who drove forward and those who remained at the headquarters. Unit commanders, NCOs, and many individual soldiers were questioned about their evaluation of their fellow soldiers' mental health status. A survey at the hospital did not report any Scud survivors reporting for sick call. On the surface, it appeared that the troops were doing their job very well, coping with the stress, and resolving any individual psychological problems on their own.

During this same period, there was contact between the chief nurse of the supporting medical group and the soldiers' brigade chaplain. All was not well with the troops, but the chaplain's attempts to reach the soldiers had been resisted. Meetings were planned and the soldiers would not show. Individual appointments with the chaplain were very limited. It was later revealed that some of the soldiers were worried that someone would label them a coward, less of a soldier, weak, or a nonworker if they took the time to be seen for counseling or to see the chaplain regarding the Scud incident.

Some just hoped their nightmares, sleepless nights, increased anger, or resentment were just part of being in Saudi, part of the war, and it would all go away when they went home. They did not feel special; they did not want to be treated like "circus performers." The Scud site had become a frequent place for Saudis and Americans to visit; the survivors resented the circus atmosphere surrounding a special monument. When the remains of the warehouse were completely removed, their resentment grew. Something that had symbolized the sacrifice of their fellow soldiers was taken away with the trash, without ceremony, only to be made into temporary living quarters for new troops. Tents were erected where the building once stood and 126 sand bags filled the "hole."

ANOTHER INTERVENTION

As the chief nurse of the Medical Group and a participant in our initial attempts to hold meetings with the survivors, I was particularly concerned about the welfare of what I considered an at risk group. When the chaplain shared his concerns with me, we proceeded to consider a new approach. As a chief nurse of the area Medical Group, I had been an active participant in planning the health care system for the troops located in the Eastern Province. All efforts in the area of communication, training, and supply had not resulted in the most timely Army medical evacuation of the wounded, getting critical medical supplies where they were needed, and prompt utilization of the triage/evacuation system. This small group of remaining survivors needed assistance in sorting out the circumstances, actions, and acts of valor performed that fateful night. This group knew valuable lessons learned for the medical planners of the future. It seemed only logical to merge the two ideas, providing valuable therapy and revealing unique medical lessons learned.

The chaplain introduced me to the key players who were each interviewed with a focus on medical "lessons learned." The company commander spent an afternoon discussing what she had done in that critical 30-minute period, arranging the experience in sequence, and gradually relating how it felt then and how it feels today. She had been experiencing frequent flashbacks to that night, usually getting the actions and circumstances all jumbled. She expressed appreciation for our conversation and said that she would encourage her unit members to see me to relate their unique experience. She also agreed to arrange for a group discussion so we could all get a clearer picture. A similar process was very successful with the quartermaster group commander and his first sergeant.

As the days progressed, the guards on duty, the radio operator, and a military policeman who had been called to the scene were all interviewed. Frequent group sessions were held focusing on the medical lessons learned as well as serving to organize the individual's and the group's experiences that night. One of the radio operators described hearing the alarms: " I went to the window to listen. Shit, they are doing it again. I can't remember them ever coming prior to the Scud heading our way. I realized that I did not have my MOPP (chemical/biological protective gear) suit with me. All of a sudden the Scud hit. I really don't remember the sound of the explosion. I was thrown to the floor inside the trailer. The desk flew across the room, almost crushing Kate [another unit member], who had luckily just moved from the desk. I could hear glass and metal coming down all around outside the trailer. My mask was gone. Kate found it. While I was putting it on, I realized I had been breathing already and threw the mask away. I said Brady [another unit member], no gas, let's go."

According to this soldier's account, Kate would stay and try to reach headquarters. The mike remained in her hand, although the radio was covered with debris. Kate had a very difficult time convincing the headquarters they had really been hit. The thought of calling for MEDEVAC did not occur, although the frequency was clearly written on both her radio (which she could no longer see) and at the headquarters. Fifteen to thirty minutes passed before the first sergeant asked Kate to call for a MEDEVAC. By this time, 8 to 10 Saudi ambulances and private vehicles were in the process of receiving the wounded from the Army soldiers who had just removed the injured from the burning building. The one opening in the wall would only permit one vehicle to pass at a time; confusion, panic, and anger prevailed. Some Saudi ambulances left with only one or two wounded. Finally, the injured were gathered in one place to expedite their prompt removal, and an additional hole was made in the wall. The dead were placed in an available Humvee to "hide the bodies."

According to these soldiers, the heroics inside the warehouse continued. The initial efforts of the radio crew were augmented by the company commander, the group commander, and a team of five from the basketball field, as well as a lieutenant, a medic, and assorted soldiers who were inside the cement barracks when the Scud hit. Masks, MOPP, and weapons were all discarded; the soldiers had one purpose in mind: "Remove their buddies from the burning, collapsing building." They could hear the sound of "exploding bullets," "feel a tracer round pass by their head" (a still unexplained experience), see flames, hear the steel girders as they moved over their heads, smell the burning food and flesh, and see parts of arms, legs, and brain with blood everywhere.

All the rescuers knew there were others attempting to remove the survivors, but no one could say who they were or what they did. It was not an effort of coordinated movement; each soldier was doing his or her very best teamed up with another available person to remove whatever they could. Each would spend 30 to 50 minutes removing bodies or body parts from within the warehouse, returning time after time without adequate lighting, walking or running right into the turmoil and fire.

The radio operator continued his description of the events:

Back in I went. I then saw a girl sitting on the floor. Her left leg was pinned under a girder. Her right thigh was torn wide open from her ass to her knee. She was holding a first aid patch to her leg. Placing my hand on her tear streaked face, "You'll be OK," I said, and went for more help. The fiberglass was in flames, all around. There was a guy lying face down on the floor. There was blood all over him. I placed my head on his back. His heart was still beating. We lifted him to a cot and carried him out. We pulled another guy out with the help of two others. Blood was running out of his back. We could not keep our hands locked together. "Hey, talk to me. I'm all right," he said. "Yeah, I know. But I'm not." After we set him down outside, I almost passed out.

After a few drags on a cigarette, I went back in to bring out more people. At one point we knew there weren't any more living. It was time for the dead. We started to pick up this one guy and half his head was gone along with his arm. There was no place to hold onto. We realized the other two guys were just standing there saying, "There's too much blood, where do we grab?" I got very mad and frustrated. "I don't give a

_____, just grab somewhere and help us." On my last sweep, I found a guy leaning against a beam in the back of the warehouse. He said he could not walk. So I helped him out of the building. Then I was assigned by the first sergeant to direct the ambulances. I don't know how many I helped. I don't want to sleep. I fear my dreams. I see them all, everyone I helped out of the warehouse and what they looked like.

One of the officers who helped remove the survivors was sent to join the group discussions but would only meet one on one. She had been experiencing nightmares, found herself outside her barracks trying to "wash her hands, to get the blood off," and had awakened in the shower in full uniform in the early morning hours. Her only peace would come during the day when she was able to accomplish her Army mission and still feel as though she was a valued member of the unit. She had been very active with the group removing bodies from the warehouse. She recalled the different people she had helped but did not feel she had done enough.

Two incidents were especially painful for her to accept and reflected her profound sense of helplessness. She was trying to assist a tall sergeant to walk. "He knew he was going to die, and I could not help him. I had no medical supplies. He just laid down and died. I could not keep him going, but he had no visible injuries." She could smell the blood and hear the moans of the wounded. The second incident occurred when she was asked to board the bus and help the wounded. Inside the bus each seat was occupied by a bleeding soldier requesting help from her and pulling on her uniform as she passed down the hallway. At the end was a soldier laying on the floor crying in agony. She recalls cradling his head on her legs as she knelt. She tried to comfort him and knew he, too, was going to die, as he did moments later.

She recalls crying and painfully leaving the bus. "I had to get out of there. I was going to be sick. I had to escape." She knew how to check wounds, apply pressure, provide comfort, and reassurance. The scene was overwhelming to her and left her with a profound sense of failure. The bus left for the hospital shortly after her experience and was the first to arrive at the local Saudi hospital—the Dhahran area trauma center. In this situation, the soldier found it helpful to revisit the scene, organize the events of the evening, and analyze the situation from the perspective of lessons learned.

Gradually she was able to identify her real contributions that night, the problem of medical supplies, and the overall confusion in the face of such a major disaster. She was starting to control her recall of the most painful events and was beginning to talk about those very events. She found remaining in Saudi, doing her job, being with the same peers, and gradually discussing the events to be healing. She knew it would be a long process but felt very hopeful about the future. She had developed some very close relationships with those who shared the events of that evening. This, too, was rewarding and would help in the healing process. She agreed to seek professional help upon redeployment.

Trucks, buses, and cars were all used at random to move the injured to hospitals. The Saudi drivers transferred most of the casualties in their ambulances to the Saudi trauma center, as designed in their civil defense plan; most were not familiar with the location of our Army hospitals. No maps were available that night, and some of our Army drivers delivered casualties to a building designed to be a hospital but actually being used as an office/housing building. These patients were then shipped by Army helicopter to an Army hospital. All the patients were at some treatment facility within 60 minutes of the attack. As best as can be determined, no lives were lost due to transportation delays or lack of available medical supplies at the scene.

A FEW CONCLUDING THOUGHTS

The process of reviewing the experiences of the soldiers the night of the Scud missile attack from a medical model perspective helped the survivors organize the events, identify their individual contributions, analyze lessons learned, resolve conflicts or feelings of failure over the events of that night, and prepare for redeployment or going home. The real process of being prepared for war and redeployment occurs as the soldier is deployed. Most of the soldiers commented that they knew what they needed to do with the survivors: check for the ABC's— is the person alive and breathing?; remove the living from the building to safety; use anything for a litter—cots, ponchos, sleeping bags, clothing, or hand carry; stop bleeding; and set up some type of triage so the most critically wounded are treated first. For the most part, the soldiers agreed they accomplished each of these tasks since they were still in control. Perimeter security, traffic control by Army military police, and lighting existed late in the disaster, allowing the Saudi civil defense system to take over and resulting in confusion, a total lack of triage, and a first come, first-served mentality. The Americans simply did not understand the Saudi system or the language.

Early intervention was initiated at the EXPO in a very nonthreatening manner. The mental health helpers were available. The immediate health needs of the soldier were met. Plans for moving forward with their mission and their accomplishments that night were identified. The composition of the intervention team was well received: chaplains, nurses, and medical personnel. Use of the same team members during the various stages of resolution was significant. The initial change in team members was not well received and proved unsuccessful, according to the soldiers. Utilizing the story telling, medical-critique method of analyzing the events was very productive in providing mental health intervention. The medics gained insight for future planning (i.e., location of medical supplies for mass casualties in the rear area, training all soldiers in basic first aid, practicing mass casualty exercises (MASCAL) for all units, and the importance of communication—early and concise). The soldiers each gained control over the events, resolved initial feelings of inadequacy, felt more comfortable seeking mental health assistance (it is hoped), and reevaluated personal security/safety issues while planning for such disasters in the future.

11

Stress Debriefings Following Death from Unexploded Ordnance

James Pecano and Deborah Hickey

INTRODUCTION

It is generally recognized that support troops are at increased risk for maladaptive combat stress reactions in time of war. In the case of medical personnel, this increased risk may be related to the fact that they are less well trained than combat troops for coping with the stressors of the combat environment. They perform a mission which, on the modern battlefield, continually exposes them to horrific human suffering and carnage, with exhausting work schedules providing little opportunity for respite. Furthermore, it has been argued that reservists are more vulnerable than active duty personnel to combat stress because reservists typically are less well prepared and trained and tend to be older, with increased personal responsibilities (Solomon, Noy, and Bar On, 1986). This is particularly relevant for the U.S. Army Medical Department given that the vast majority of combat-deployable medical assets are reserve units.

Certain protective factors, identified from previous military conflicts and incorporated into current Army combat stress doctrine, can be expected to provide some buffering of combat stress for medical personnel. Such protective factors include high unit cohesion and morale; effective, competent leadership; tough, realistic training; as well as individual competence and fitness (Noy, Nardi, and Solomon, 1986; Belenky, 1987).

While serving as mental health officers with a combat stress control team during the Gulf War, we were called on to debrief a medical company which had sustained significant casualties in two separate incidents, resulting in the deaths of two unit members—a physician and a medic. In this chapter, we present findings from our experience to illustrate the potential vulnerabilities of medical personnel to combat stress. We also demonstrate the importance of unit protective factors, such as cohesion and effective leadership (in both insulating unit members from the effects of combat stress and facilitating adaptation after extremely traumatic events). Finally, we highlight the importance of conducting prompt critical incident stress debriefings in the combat zone.

BACKGROUND

On February 28, 1991, a convoy of members of one medical platoon from the 142nd Medical Clearing Company and some British medical personnel set forth on a mission to augment the medical assets of the Main Support Battalion of the 1st Infantry Division in Iraq. In midmorning, the forward movement was stopped when the lead vehicles encountered what were believed to be Iraqi soldiers surrendering to the American medical platoon. Shortly after the convoy stopped, the sound of an explosion was heard. It immediately became apparent that one of the vehicles had been involved. A physician who was riding in the vehicle was killed, and three other passengers suffered serious injuries. During the resulting confusion, the immediate impression was that the convoy was under attack. The response was to dismount and assume firing positions in the sands surrounding the vehicles. Shortly thereafter, the sounds of a second explosion and the screams of a young female were heard. It was assumed she had been injured as a result of enemy fire or accidental detonation of a buried enemy land mine. A nearby British soldier also sustained minor wounds.

The reactions of other soldiers varied from an instinct to pursue the believed enemy into the sandy hills, to a state of immobilization, confusion, and fear, to a recognition of the need to attempt to leave the area as quickly as possible. Along with all these feelings, there was the need to provide immediate medical care for the wounded.

At the time of these events, a sandstorm had begun. It severely impaired visibility, thereby impairing vision of the hills from which the attack had been perceived and delaying any attempts at evacuating the wounded via air ambulance. The young female medic was dragged to safety and placed into a nearby ambulance. She was ultimately evacuated by helicopter to a combat support hospital, where she died from her wounds.

Unit members initially believed that the vehicle accidentally detonated an enemy land mine. A second mine apparently detonated when the female medic inadvertently rolled over onto it. This was soon to become suspect by some members of the unit, who had inspected the vehicle and found the chassis intact with a hole in the floor which appeared to be a point of exit rather than a point of entrance. Some unit members believed that the pattern of shattered windows was consistent with that of an RPG (rocket-propelled grenade) which entered from the left passenger window and resulted in an explosion of glass outward in the rear of the vehicle.

Five days after this incident, the unit experienced a second tragedy while established in a tactical assembly area. A fierce storm developed which caused the power generators to fail. An enlisted medic reached under his cot to obtain a flashlight. Suddenly, an explosion was heard. The medic sustained significant injury to his shoulder and arm. Nearby, a female soldier lay unconscious and was presumed dead. A third female occupant sustained significant facial injuries. Upon removing the injured from the tent, it was discovered that the female medic was, in fact, alive although comatose and in respiratory arrest. These injured soldiers were immediately evacuated to a nearby combat support hospital, where they were treated and evacuated to Germany for more definitive medical care.

The immediate response by the unit was fear that they were again under attack. Ultimately, it became evident that cluster bomblets had been responsible for this explosion, and that various members of the unit had accumulated bomblets as war souvenirs. This was done in ignorance of the true nature of the objects, as members later stated that they originally believed them to be spent Iraqi flares which were safe to possess.

Within a few days, the remaining unit members were reunited with the medical company. They experienced a confusing array of reactions as other unit members struggled to come to terms with the loss of their comrades and make sense out of their experiences. The members of the unit became quite divided. Official accounts listed the initial casualties as resulting from land mine detonation. While some accepted this, many came to question this in light of the second incident and amid accusations that one officer in the unit had encouraged the collection of the bomblets by misidentifying them as spent Iraqi flare caps. Others continued to maintain that the convoy had been attacked.

Over the next week, the medical company became extremely dysfunctional, and the commanding officer, persuaded by several of the physicians in the unit, requested that a psychiatric team intervene. A team comprised of a psychiatrist, clinical psychologist, and clinical social worker was dispatched to debrief the unit.

CRITICAL INCIDENTS STRESS DEBRIEFING

The importance of early intervention and debriefing after disasters has been well established in the civilian literature (Mitchell, 1983; Mitchell and Bray, 1990) and is incorporated into U.S. Army combat stress control doctrine. The ultimate objective of the debriefing process is to provide participants the opportunity to assimilate the traumatic event into their experience, thereby reducing the anxiety and distress associated with the event and facilitating recovery from the trauma. The process provides participants with an opportunity to ventilate their emotional reactions to the event, to gain a more complete view of the experience by filling missing or incomplete information and correcting misperceptions, and to understand the expected psychological reactions to traumatic events, thereby normalizing emotional experiences. The debriefing is typically held soon after the traumatic experience to facilitate effective adaptation and prevent symptoms from taking hold and psychologically disabling the individual. Optimally, all individuals involved in the trauma should be present at the debriefing, which is best conducted in a group format with groups comprised of individuals with similar experiences of the trauma.

Our first goal in the debriefing process was to gain the support of the unit chain of command. We attended the commander's staff meeting, during which we were introduced and our purpose was clarified. We gathered important information about the leaders' perceptions of problems within the unit and their assessment of the unit's adaptive functioning. It was clear that the leadership recognized the enormous stress and the difficulties unit members were having. They welcomed our consultation but were unwilling to mandate involvement for all unit members in the debriefings. Because the unit had been divided into individual platoons, and because each of the platoons differentially experienced the trauma, we decided to preserve that integrity in the debriefing process.

Overall, we conducted five separate debriefings: each of the three medical platoons, the headquarters platoon, and a separate debriefing for the chain of command. The debriefings were relatively structured. We introduced the debriefing as an opportunity for members to discuss their feelings around the events which had occurred. We related our understanding of the facts as we knew them in an effort to stimulate the group to relate their perceptions and experiences. When appropriate, we focused on clarifying misperceptions and examined alternative explanations. We took the opportunity to educate the groups about the psychological processes involved in adapting to trauma and the range of expected symptoms and feelings. Finally, we made ourselves available for individual consultation for those who desired to meet with us privately.

Approximately 60 percent of the unit members participated in the group debriefings. In addition, we provided follow up individual care for 18 individuals who were experiencing significant symptomatology requiring more tailored intervention. Our intervention with the unit lasted three weeks.

FINDINGS AND ANALYSIS

Our findings are organized according to content areas, which emerged naturally from the debriefings but which are known to be significant in combat stress control. It was difficult to characterize the unit's overall adaptation to the events experienced, as the experiences of the events were so different among unit members. Nevertheless, the unit was quite fragmented and dysfunctional. In addition to the difficulties unit members were experiencing related to the two ordnance incidents, they were also struggling to adapt to the theater wide stressors associated with the cessation of combat operations and redeployment back to the United States.   Nevertheless, our assessment was that many individuals were stuck in the adaptive process. They were well aware that many of the feelings and reactions they were experiencing were in response to the trauma.   Yet they seemed unable to integrate their experiences and were struggling to find a positive way to resolve conflictual issues that had emerged as a result of the incidents.

Lack of Information

One of the key issues impeding the adaptive process was the ambiguous and conflicting accounts, official and unofficial, of the incidents.   This generated different realities of the experience and served to impair coherent integration of the trauma.   The different official and unofficial accounts generated a division among unit members with a shared paranoia around two disparate sets of beliefs, which served to reconcile conflicting internal and external realities.

The common belief was that the Army was now engaged in a massive cover up of the facts surrounding the initial incident which resulted in the two deaths. One view held that the Army leadership realized that it had erred in sending a medical unit into hostile territory with inadequate security and means to protect itself.   As a result, it had been attacked by Iraqi soldiers feigning surrender. According to this view, the Army was now engaged in a massive cover up to avoid the negative publicity which could result by holding that the deaths were the result of land mines.

A second set of beliefs evolved from individuals who had inspected the vehicle and had suspected that the explosion had originated inside the vehicle. For this group of individuals, the cover up served to protect a senior ranking officer from the unit, who was said to have misidentified the ordnance and encouraged its collection as souvenirs.   Its subsequent detonation had resulted in the two deaths.   Both sets of beliefs served to deepen a sense of distrust in the leadership of the unit.

In our opinion, the genesis of this phenomenon was related to the inherent ambiguity and complexity of officially determining exactly what had occurred in a timely manner.   It appeared to be more directly attributed to the failure on the part of the chain of command to communicate accurate information rapidly to unit members as it became available.   Although information that the deaths were probably not combat related in the strict sense brought forth a host of new emotional reactions, these seemed to be more readily processed by the unit members.

Morale and Cohesion

Unit members generally agreed that prior to the deployment of the unit to Southwest Asia, cohesion and morale were high within the medical company. Many unit members had drilled with this unit for significant periods of time, and training was usually conducted in a manner which preserved the integrity of the company as a whole. As a result, the members of the unit generally felt close to one another. However, 40 of the 142 members of the unit were cross leveled (moved from another unit for fill a specific position that was vacant) into the company at the time it was mobilized to bring it to strength for deployment. Thus, there was little time to integrate these new members adequately into the unit, and the cohesion was weakened.

Medical planning within the theater emphasized modular and flexible deployment of medical assets as needed. The unit was divided in order to meet the different missions assigned to the company. Generally, each detachment from the unit was assigned to augment existing medical units. As a result of this fragmentation, there was a further disruption in cohesion as unit members struggled to establish a collective identity in terms of the detachments to which they were assigned. An unhealthy competitiveness between the detachments evolved within the theater and even reached the point of detachment members stealing supplies from one another.

The breakdown in cohesion was even more problematic in that detachment members experienced significant difficulty integrating into the medical units to which they were assigned. Part of this was simply a function of the lack of time to assimilate adequately into a new unit prior to the initiation of ground combat operations. There was a more pernicious process which interfered with effective integration into the gaining units. Unit members described feeling "looked down upon" (as reservists) by members of the regular Army units which they augmented. Their perception was one of second-class citizenship and an unacceptance of them and unwillingness to integrate them into the existing unit. Fortunately, the eminent success of combat operations resulted in extremely light American casualties. Ironically, though, this resulted in a much more limited medical mission and, in a sense, restricted the opportunities for team building and integration among augmented medical personnel through performance of their duties.

The breakdown in cohesion experienced by the members of this unit placed them at increased risk for maladaptive combat stress reactions. The divisiveness fostered projection of blame, splitting the unit into "good and bad" platoons and "officers and enlisted." This breakdown in cohesion hampered effective adaptation to the trauma afterward by reducing the availability of social support: a coping strategy afforded by high unit cohesion.

Leadership and Training

One of the most significant issues that emerged from our debriefings was that the leadership of the unit was not perceived as effective and competent. This seemed to emanate from the fact that 11 of the 14 officers in the unit were cross leveled into the company upon activation of the unit to bring it to strength for deployment.   The officers (mostly physicians) were from the Individual Ready Reserve, and while most were seen as technically competent in their professional skills, they were perceived as militarily inexperienced and unskilled.   This served to create a schism between the officers and enlisted which contributed to lack of confidence in the leadership.   This schism was widened by the creation of a confusing leadership position called the platoon commander, who was the highest ranking physician in the platoon. This created ambiguity and lack of continuity in the platoon chain of command and served to undermine the authority and effectiveness of the platoon leaders.

We encountered an extreme sense of entitlement among some of the officers coupled with a disrespect for the enlisted soldiers.   This was manifested in double standards which existed regarding theater policies and privileges (e.g., phones, showers, uniforms) and a failure for many of the officers to set an example in standards of behavior.   We primarily attributed this to inadequate leadership training and experience of the medical officers involved. Nevertheless, such attitudes served to erode morale and weaken confidence in the leadership.

Related to the issues of leadership and military training was the reportedly poor preparation in combat related military skills identified by members of the unit.   These included identifying military ordnance, processing POWs, and maneuvering in hostile territory. Many unit members felt that this was primarily responsible for the occurrence of the two incidents.

The perceived ineffectiveness of the leadership led to a   projection of culpability onto the leaders for the incidents and casualties. This compromised the leaders' usual capacity to assist unit members in their adaptation to combat stress. The inability of the leadership to intervene earlier was also related to the fact that two key and respected members of the leadership were themselves casualties, both from this experience and as a product of previous combat experience.

Combat Stress Reactions

Many unit members were experiencing common symptoms and reactions associated with traumatic experience. Unit members most closely involved in the two incidents related a range of symptoms, including nightmares and sleep disturbance, intrusive thoughts and images, depression and crying spells, anxiety and hyperarousal, fear of the dark, irritability, and guilt.   Many individuals were relieved to learn that their symptoms were normal, expected responses to trauma which could be expected to improve. The value of education, even with medical personnel who might be assumed to be more psychologically sophisticated than usual, proved essential.

In addition, we were able to identify a number of individuals who required more intensive intervention. Most required only one or two individual sessions with one of us. Some required more extensive treatment. Several individuals experienced an exacerbation of underlying posttraumatic stress from previous combat experience. Two individuals required adjunctive pharmacological treatment for their symptoms. We treated all individuals with strict adherence to the sound practices of combat stress control doctrine, and especially with the clear expectation that they would fully recover and return to duty.

DISCUSSION

Although the experiences of this unit in Operation Desert Storm were atypical for a medical unit, we believe that our findings revealed factors which may not be unique to this unit and which can contribute to the vulnerability of medical personnel to maladaptive combat stress reactions. Combat stress control doctrine has well emphasized the importance of effective leadership, unit cohesion, and morale as buffers against deleterious responses to combat stress. These are actively developed and sustained in combat arms units. As a rule, medical personnel tend to be less identified with their military role compared to their professional role. Consequently, less attention is paid to developing military and leadership skills. By virtue of the structure of medical units in time of war, medical officers are thrust into key leadership and command roles. Some may lack the preparation, experience, or effective leadership style to assume these roles. Conflicts within the chain of command can develop when allegiance is given to individuals with perceived authority rather than legitimate authority. The importance of developing and maintaining cohesion and morale in a medical unit may pale in comparison to the exigencies of medical preparation and planning in time of war. There is no substitute for effective leadership, especially in time of war, and this must be developed in medical officers as much as in officers in the combat arms.

Whether due to inadequate monitoring of reserve unit strengths prior to the mobilization or to the inherent staffing difficulties generated by a massive medical mobilization, it was apparent that the extensive cross leveling of personnel into medical units prior to their deployment contributed to a disruption in cohesiveness and unit integrity. The medical company we debriefed was not unusual in this regard. Although we recognize the need for flexible, modular deployment of medical assets on the modern battlefield, we are convinced that it worked against the establishment and maintenance of unit cohesion and weakened its protective and healing potential.

Finally, our experience validates the necessity for timely, effective debriefing for all military units in combat operations regardless of the nature of the trauma. This is an important function of mental health officers in combat stress control doctrine. Surprisingly, few in our detachment were familiar with the process of conducting debriefings. This must be rectified if mental health officers are to be effective in combat stress control and casualty care.

We are aware that some may take exception to our conceptualization of the issues and reactions we encountered under the rubric of combat stress. We contend that the stimuli for the difficulties we encountered were a product of the tactical situation and military environment typical for a medical unit. Moreover, isolated, infrequent incidents such as the ones we described may be the primary source of combat stress for noncombatants on the battlefield in future rapid, highly mobile, and highly lethal conflicts, as well as in military operations short of war. More importantly, we believe that framing the issues from this perspective greatly facilitates appropriate unit and individual intervention.

REFERENCES

Belenky, G. (1987). "Varieties of reaction and adaptation to combat experience." In W. Menninger (ed.), *Military Psychiatry: Learning from Experience*. Topeka, Kan: The Menninger Foundation, 64–79.

Mitchell, J. T. (1983). "When disaster strikes: The critical incidents stress debriefing process." *J. of Emergency Med. Serv.*, January, 36–39.

Mitchell, J. T. and G. Bray. (1990*). Emergency Services Stress: Guidelines For Preserving The Health And Careers Of Emergency Services Personnel*. Englewood Cliffs, N.J.: Prentice Hall.

Noy, S., C. Nardi and Z. Solomon. (1986). "Battle and military unit characteristics and the prevalence of psychiatric casualties." In N.A. Milgram (ed.), *Stress and Coping in Time of War*. New York: Brunner/Mazel, 73–77.

Solomon, Z., S. Noy and R. Bar On. (1986). "Who is at high risk for a combat stress reaction syndrome?" In N.A. Milgram (ed.), *Stress and Coping in Time of War*. New York: Brunner/Mazel, 78–83.

12

Rapid Interventions after a Disaster at Sea

Michael P. Dinneen

INTRODUCTION

This chapter describes a wartime naval accident which directly and powerfully affected two very different crews. The account is used to highlight a variety of combat mental health issues associated with the Gulf War.

BACKGROUND

The U.S. Navy hospital ship *Comfort* was deployed to the Persian Gulf region in support of the Gulf War combat operation. The ship was designed with 12 operating rooms and a maximum capacity of 1000 beds, including 100 beds for intensive care, 280 for intermediate care, 120 for light care, and 500 for limited care. When fully staffed, the ship has a crew of 1200 and functions as a small independent city. It is also one of the world's largest hospitals—on land or sea.

The *Comfort's* crews shared with other sailors deployed in the Gulf waters the common stressors associated with life at sea in a hostile fire zone. The ship had been deployed for several months in response to the Iraqi invasion of Kuwait in August 1990. By October of that year, the strain of isolation, cramped quarters, lack of privacy, and the contradictory fear and boredom were taking their toll on the morale of the ship's crew. An added stress factor was the fact that the *Comfort* was on its first operational deployment. After being converted from its original configuration as an oil tanker, the *Comfort* lay relatively dormant for several years. It had never deployed, and its capabilities had never been tested. In addition, the vast majority of the crew was also inexperienced with sea and with war and lacked burn/trauma experience.

On August 9, 1990, just seven days after Iraq had invaded Kuwait, the crew of the *Comfort* was notified that they would be deploying in support of Coalition Forces. This notification was the beginning of an eight-month odyssey wherein men and women from disparate backgrounds were brought together with less than a week's notice and sent to sea to face an imminent war. The *Comfort* arrived in the Kuwaiti theater of operations on September 6, 1990 with only 500 of its designed 1000 beds ready and operational.

While there is an extensive literature on soldier stress issues, there is surprisingly little written about the psychological effects on naval crew members during a rapid deployment, or psychological issues during naval deployments in general. Personal accounts by psychiatrists from prior hospital ship deployments have described the number and diagnoses of psychiatric casualties brought to the ship for care but have not commented on the crew's or their own adaptation (Strange and Arthur, 1967). In the single available personal account by a hospital ship psychiatrist, Dr. Morgan O'Connell of the British Royal Navy admits to spending nearly two years attempting to write about his experience during the Falklands War and states, "The delay may well be a reflection of my own problems."

The situation that the crew of the *Comfort* faced was what some have termed "the immediate precrisis period" (Mitchell, 1986). This is the period when a person knows that there maybe a disaster or crisis at any moment and yet does not know how extensive or serious the crisis will be. Like other sailors deployed to the Gulf, the crew of the *Comfort* faced five months of precrisis stress during the period of Gulf War air and ground operations. The atmosphere on board the *Comfort* was characterized by tension, anxiety, boredom, heightened awareness, unpredictability, and radically altered personal and professional roles (naval medical personnel who left their comfortable hospitals for a strange and difficult shipboard environment).

The *Comfort*'s 45 member mental health team quickly determined that it would not only have to establish services for combat stress casualties during war, but it would also have to establish a mental health service for noncombat care, including mental health services for the *Comfort*'s crew. If, however, the ship received large numbers of psychiatric casualties, it was clear that the ship's mental health staff would be busy taking care of casualties and the crew of the *Comfort* would need to be prepared to provide much of their own psychological support.

The mental health team identified its initial task as providing information and training to the *Comfort*'s crew as prophylaxis against combat stress. The concept that overwhelming stress would produce emotional turmoil and decompensation in susceptible individuals or groups was the guiding principle in the plan for health promotion activities on the *Comfort*. If the stress became powerful enough, any crew member might become overwhelmed and ultimately, with the loss of key crew members, the ship would not be able to accomplish its mission. If the stress acting on the group could be lessened, then the crew would be able to function more effectively and with greater stamina.

The mental health team also recognized that the ship's crew is a closed social system with a normally strong internal structure wherein each crew member relies on his or her shipmate for survival (Weisaeth et al., 1986). The *Comfort* was naturally divided into work spaces; most wards had a staff of 20 to 30 nurses and corpsmen. Other work spaces, administrative areas, and support facilities were composed of groups of 20 to 40 individuals that functioned as teams. Promoting group cohesiveness in these teams was viewed as the primary initial goal of the mental health team. Through these groups, the mental health team developed a trauma staff skilled not only in techniques of physiologic treatment, but also in social and psychological care of their patients and themselves. Initially, a majority of the ship's crew received two one-hour lectures covering basic stress management and care of the combat casualty. These were didactic presentations followed by group discussion and were given at work centers to 20 to 30 individuals at a time.

Four lessons were conveyed repeatedly during these sessions: You cannot provide care to casualties unless you have cared for yourselves; your primary support will come from the team that you build together; you will provide a tremendous service to the people you treat if you listen to their accounts of their experiences, their war stories; and finally, you will survive this experience and perhaps even prosper from it if you speak with your friends about what you are seeing, hearing, touching, smelling, and feeling.

Much of the initial training in stress management and care of the combat casualty was targeted at nurses and corpsmen because those individuals were considered to be at high risk for acute and chronic posttraumatic stress disorder (PTSD) (Norman, 1986). Many years after the Vietnam conflict, several studies documented a high incidence of PTSD among military nurses (Norman, 1986; Baker, 1989). Navy nurses typically possess superior clinical skills, but they often serve primarily as supervisors, mentors, teachers, disciplinarians, and surrogate parents for young corpsmen (Shiffer, 1990). In a stirring account of her experiences in Vietnam, Rear Admiral Frances Shea described how she was called on to become a "substitute mother, wife, lover, sister—the shoulder to cry on." She went on to say, however, that nurses "would not share with anyone" their own trauma. They simply "toughed it out" and paid the consequences later (Shea, 1983).

Many of the corpsmen assigned to the *Comfort* were recent graduates of Navy basic medical training programs and had little or no clinical experience. Of the approximately 25 corpsmen assigned to the psychiatric wards, only eight had prior experience in mental health care. These young men and women had no way to know how they would do if they were called on to treat catastrophic casualties.

The mental health team conceptualized for the crew the fact that the trauma of deployment and shipboard life in a war zone is an abnormal stressor that caused normal people to have expectable, normal reactions. This simplified model of psychological response to trauma was accepted by the crew and assuaged people's anxiety when they recognized that they were eating poorly, sleeping fitfully, snapping at their friends, or having nightmares. People actually began to report spontaneously when their symptoms subsided. This gave hope to other crew members who were adapting more slowly. The message was conveyed that if the ship received mass casualties, it would be even more important to practice regular informal group debriefings.

PREPARATIONS FOR RAPID INTERVENTIONS

After the initial combat stress management lectures were completed, advanced training in critical incident stress debriefing (CISD) was provided to 56 members of the ship's crew (representing all the clinical and support departments). This eight hour seminar provided a cadre of trained individuals with the skills and knowledge required to "help the helpers" in the event of critical incidents occurring aboard ship. One of the participants in the training was a nurse who had been stationed aboard the U.S.S. *Repose* during the Vietnam conflict. She explained to the class how her inability to tell friends or colleagues about her experiences had contributed to her becoming isolated and withdrawn after the war. Her endorsement of regular group debriefing during continuous trauma lent tremendous credence to the seminar.

One of the tenets of combat psychiatry is that mental health workers should be available to travel to the front lines to provide assistance and consultation. In practice, this is difficult because it requires that mental health workers abandon the relatively protected hospital environment and travel to an unknown and potentially hostile environment. In addition, workers must assume an altered identity as consultant, planner, teacher, and advocate. Speaking skills and one's power of persuasion become critically important and must be combined with a clear understanding of military mission priorities. The Navy established Special Psychiatric Rapid Intervention Teams (SPRINTs) in 1977 following the observation that shipboard disasters aboard the U.S.S. *Belknap* and U.S.S. *Kennedy* in 1975 and the U.S.S. *Guam* and U.S.S. *Trenton* in 1977 had resulted in long term problems, including increased psychiatric disability, poor work performance, marital discord, and psychiatric hospitalization (McCaughey, 1987).

SPRINT employs techniques developed by combat psychiatrists during World War I and World War II to provide aggressive psychological support to service members traumatized by disaster. The team's effectiveness is enhanced by its availability for immediate deployment and adaptability to a variety of situations. The team's goal is to provide crisis intervention, group debriefings, and command consultation which would catalyze the normal process of recovery from psychological trauma. The team is meant to temporarily augment and permanently strengthen existing support systems.

A CRITICAL INCIDENT STRESS RESPONSE

The naval vessel the U.S.S. *Iwo Jima* carried a Marine Corps Battalion Landing Team and its equipment for air amphibious assaults. The *Iwo Jima* was commissioned in 1961 and is part of the U.S. Atlantic fleet. Its crew of 609 was joined by 1746 embarked Marines. It is a large industrial complex which includes what may be thought of as a floating airport.

The *Iwo Jima* had completed several demanding overseas deployments before being ordered to proceed to the Persian Gulf in support of the first phase of the Gulf War named Operation Desert Shield. On October 30, 1990, the *Iwo Jima* was steaming out of a Bahrain port after completing boiler repairs. The crew was somewhat anxious because the ship had recently experienced a series of mechanical failures. The boiler had been pressurized for the first time since repairs were completed, and the night crew had just been relieved.

A fresh crew had assumed duty in the boiler room when steam began to escape suddenly from one of the main valves connecting the boiler to the turbine. Only one man was able to scamper uninjured up the ladder to safety. Within seconds, the entire boiler room filled with superheated steam, scalding the remaining 10 men. The ship went to general quarters, power was lost, and the medical and damage control teams went into action. Six of the ten scalded men died in the boiler room. The other four men managed somehow to climb the ladders out of the boiler room into the crew's mess deck, screaming in agony. Their friends attempted to render aid. One sailor said later that he could not recognize one of the victims, a close friend, because the swelling and discoloration caused by the steam burns was so disfiguring.

Survivors were gasping for air as their wind pipes swelled shut. They had to be intubated on the floor of the mess deck. While trying to move their friends, litter bearers could not avoid pulling off large pieces of skin. While the four men were being stabilized in the medical department, the *Comfort* was notified of the disaster. These four survivors were then flown by helicopter to the *Comfort*. Once the patients arrived on board the *Comfort*, there were two ships that had been traumatized by the boiler explosion: the *Iwo Jima*, where the accident had occurred, and the *Comfort*, where the critically injured survivors had been evacuated.

We will first describe the assistance rendered aboard the *Iwo Jima* and then describe the care provided for the crew members of the *Comfort*.

The *Comfort* had received word of the disaster 90 minutes before the casualties arrived. Several of the members of the mental health team had served on SPRINTs and saw the opportunity to render assistance to the crew of the *Iwo*

Jima. The commanding officer of the *Comfort*, a psychiatrist, agreed that a psychological debriefing team should be sent to assist the *Iwo Jima* crew. This was not an easy decision because sending a team meant that a significant portion of the *Comfort*'s mental health personnel would be temporarily lost at a time when war was potentially imminent.

SPRINT ACTIVITIES ON BOARD THE *IWO JIMA*

Arrangements for transportation were hastily made, and the ship's psychiatrist left by helicopter about four hours after the explosion. He arrived in Bahrain several hours later. The *Iwo Jima* was tied to the pier but had lost electrical power. The ship was quiet, hot, and filled with a pervasive odor. The psychiatrist was met by the ship's doctor and escorted to meet with the commanding officer (CO). The tragedy was discussed in detail, and the commanding officer gave permission for a psychological debriefing of crew members.

During the initial meeting, the psychiatrist had the opportunity to advise the commanding officer to keep the crew on board ship (and not offer a shore liberty), to establish phone services for the crew, and to ensure frequent overhead announcements informing the crew of any developments. The CO quickly implemented most of the psychiatrist's suggestions. In addition, assuring proper rest and nutrition were emphasized as ways to limit stress reactions. After the meeting, the psychiatrist requested that a psychologist and two hospital corpsmen be sent from the *Comfort* to join the debriefing team.

The ship's executive office (XO) then conducted a tour of the boiler room. The entire room was shrouded in the white remains of the halon used in fire fighting, which gave the dark space an eerie feel. The pervasive odor was intense in the room. Pieces of skin remained on walkways and ladders, and one crew member's boot was lodged among some machinery. The XO educated the psychiatrist about the accident and also about the ship. He then worked with the psychiatrist to identify groups of sailors at risk for stress reactions and planned a schedule of debriefings.

Next, the psychiatrist met with the ship's chaplains, a psychiatric nurse, and some other members of the ship's augmented medical department. Again, practical suggestions concerning early interventions and more information about the accident and about the ship were exchanged between the psychiatrist and the crew. Finally, several hours were spent educating the ship's medical providers and chaplains about crisis debriefing and expectable responses to emotional trauma.

Several principles guided the initial approach to the intervention. First, the psychiatrist did not leave the *Comfort* until he had received an invitation from the CO of the *Iwo Jima*. This ensured that the psychiatrist arrived as an invited guest, not a suspect intruder. Second, a comprehensive picture of the trauma was constructed before group debriefings were conducted. The stance, "I am a consultant, please educate me" worked very well. Third, the recipients of aid were assured that help would be practical and reasonable. Brief, concrete suggestions that prevented secondary trauma or exhaustion built credibility. The crew of the *Iwo Jima* needed to know that the SPRINT team was promoting a healthy response to trauma, not searching for weakness, sickness, or scapegoats.

The second day of the intervention began at 0700 with a briefing for the CO and department heads. This provided an opportunity to explain to the ship's leaders the purpose of SPRINT interventions in general and the specific plan for the *Iwo Jima* intervention. Immediately thereafter, all of the ship's officers were assembled in small groups for a lecture on crisis response and the likely sequelae of the disaster. At each session, the message was clear: The crew of the *Iwo Jima* was a group of normal people who could be expected to have normal and predictable responses to a grossly abnormal stressor.

Formal debriefings for 20 to 30 individuals at a time began at 9 in the morning. Group debriefings were conducted continuously for 15 hours; over 350 crew members were seen. Two teams of facilitators worked simultaneously and met between groups to discuss. progress and problems. Group composition was based on the sailors' normal working relationships within work spaces. Attendance was mandatory. The members at greatest risk were judged to be those who had been on fire fighting teams, handled dead or dying sailors, or who had worked in the boiler spaces. The debriefings, which lasted about 90 minutes, were structured but allowed the open expression of thoughts and feelings about the disaster.

Group members were asked to describe their experiences during the steam explosion. This allowed the members to construct a coherent picture of the disaster. It was clear that in the midst of confusion, heat, blackness, and terror, the sailors had not been able to comprehend the big picture. During this part of the debriefing, myths were constructively shattered.

Next, people's thoughts and reactions concerning the tragedy were elicited. This naturally led to the expression of strong feelings. Many of the sailors had clung to the belief that they could have prevented the tragedy somehow or saved one of their shipmates. The sharing of information allowed them to see that this simply was not so. Crew members feeling the most anguish were comforted by their friends. Anger was frighteningly intense and was often directed at the group facilitators or other authority figures. Many of the men volunteered that they were not sleeping or that they were avoiding sleep to prevent nightmares. One of the sleeping quarters had become a symbol of the loss because several of the bunks were conspicuously empty.

The expression of thoughts, feelings, and reactions promoted an awakening to the shared experience. This was reinforced and given structure when group facilitators explained in detail that the crew's emotional, physical, cognitive, and behavioral symptoms were normal responses to the tragedy. Finally, crew members were advised to avoid alcohol, fistfights, and major life decisions until the impact of the immediate trauma had subsided.

After the last session, all of the debriefers met to discuss and digest the day's events. The following day, the team was asked to provide lectures on the crisis response to the Marines that were on the ship. These lectures were delivered by a hospital corpsman on the flight deck. The team then attended a formal memorial service for the deceased sailors, outbriefed the CO, planned for follow up services with the ship's medical department, and departed. The entire intervention lasted two days.

CRITICAL CARE ABOARD THE *COMFORT*

The *Iwo Jima* disaster had a profound effect on the crew of the *Comfort* as well. When word of the casualties was received, the burn unit on the *Comfort* was decorated as a haunted house in preparation for Halloween. Within hours, a room that had been prepared for a party was converted back to an intensive care unit. The four *Iwo Jima* victims had burns over 90 percent of their bodies. Many of the staff members in the ICU had never seen such catastrophic burns. Over the next 13 hours, the medical staff struggled to save the burn victims, but they all died.

There was sadness and some sense of demoralization even though the senior physicians repeatedly explained that burns of that severity were inevitably fatal. There was an obvious breach in the defenses of denial, which some crew members had continued to use effectively. *Comfort* crew members had friends aboard the *Iwo Jima*, including among the casualties. The dangers of life at sea, even in the absence of hostilities, were more difficult to ignore.

As the patients were moved through the patient flow route of the *Comfort*, staff who had been taking care of them earlier were provided status reports. The *Comfort*'s staff wanted to know not only about the clinical conditions but also whatever had been learned about their identities as well as the condition of the *Iwo Jima* and the remaining crew. Members of the mental health team gathered this information and presented it in these early large group informational briefings.

Later, with coordination by the senior psychiatric nurse and the social worker, a number of crew members who had attended the critical incident stress debriefing seminar cofacilitated several debriefing sessions for the *Comfort* staff (provided separately for each medical sectionion). The objectives and techniques used for the debriefings aboard *Comfort* followed closely the model used aboard *Iwo Jima*. Strong anger was expressed over issues such as the unit supervisors requiring stress debriefings, the presence of visitors and cameras in the unit, and selection of who was to care for the casualties and who was to speak to the media. Although some people were reluctant to speak at first, they slowly revealed their sadness, feelings of helplessness, and fear that the *Iwo*

Jima casualties were a harbinger of things to come. Many people had not been prepared for the horror of watching helplessly as sailors died.

After the formal debriefings, the crew's attention shifted to the question of whether the previously planned Halloween parties would be permitted. That decision was delegated to the staff of the critical care units who had planned to host the event. Most of them had also been directly involved in the care of the casualties. Having been formally debriefed, they continued the recovery by solving the problem of whether or not to redecorate the haunted house and proceed with the Halloween party. After much deliberation, the staff reached the conclusion that the party should and would go on.

That evening there was a fantastic house of horrors aboard ship. Most members of the crew wore realistically gory "costumes," which included the moulage they had perfected during mass casualty drills. Benign or glamorous costumes were noticeably absent. Taps was postponed at the hour for lights out when a long line remained of people who still wanted to go through the house of horrors. At the end of the line was the commanding officer. After he went through, Taps was sounded. Although no such interpretations were made explicit, it was a most unusual and effective memorial. The next day, the crew resumed routine operations with increased confidence and sense of purpose.

Six weeks later, eight soldiers were brought to the *Comfort* nearly comatose after they had accidentally ingested methanol. The medical staff responded immediately, providing superior care and allowing all of the patients to recover without any long-term sequelae. That successful experience established a tremendous amount of confidence.

CONCLUSION

Twelve months after the explosion on the *Iwo Jima*, in reflecting on these events and the meanings she has attached to them, one nurse would recall that the experience was "burned in my mind. The critical incident stress debriefing training was great to have had before it was needed." Another nurse attributed meaning to the event: "It came at a good time for us in a way. It brought the reality of the situation to the younger staff. Caring for the expectant (those expected to die) broke through the denial of what war might be like. It was in a way a good thing for us to go through before the war."

During the five months following the steam explosion, no crew member from the *Iwo Jima* was psychiatrically hospitalized for reasons related to the disaster. The ship was repaired and completed its mission in support of the Gulf War. The ship's doctor reported that people continued to speak about their losses, their anger, and their fears of another accident, but they did their jobs and supported one another. Over time, the group's grief became less intense.

REFERENCES

Baker, R. R. (1989). "The military nurse experience in Vietnam: Stress and impact." *J. of Clin. Psychol.*, 45:736–744.

Becker, D. J., et al. (1991). *A Gas Mask Desensitization Program for Sailors in a War Zone*. Presented at the 1991 AMSUS Convention, New York.

Glass, A. J. (1955). "Principles of combat psychiatry." *Mil. Med.*, 117:27–33.

McCaughey, B. G. (1987). "U.S. Navy special psychiatric rapid intervention team." *Mil. Med.*, 152:133–135.

Mitchell, J. T. (1986). "Assessing and managing the psychological impact of terrorism, civil disorder, disasters, and mass casualties." *Emergency Care Q.*, 2(1):51–58.

Moore, J. (ed). (1984). *Jane's Fighting Ships*. London: Janes Publishing Co., Ltd.

Norman, E. M. (1986). "A study of female military nurses in Vietnam during the war years 1965–1973." *J. of Nursing Hist.*, 2(1):43–60.

O'Connell, M. R. (1986). "Stress-induced stress in the psychiatrist: A naval psychiatrist's personal view of the Falklands' conflict." *Stress Med.*, 2:307–314.

Shea, F. T. (1983). "Stress of caring for combat casualties." *U.S. Navy Med.*, 74:4–7.

Shiffer, S. W. (1990). "Today's role of the Navy nurse." *Mil. Med.*, 155(5):208–213.

Strange, R. E. and R. J. Arthur. (1967). "Hospital ship psychiatry in a war zone." *Amer. J. Psychiat.*, 124(3):281–286.

Weisaeth, L., P. Gorm and M. van Overloop. (1986, September). *Naval Combat Stress-Reactions*. Presented to NATO Conference on Disasters, Paris, France.

13

Occupational Therapy and the Treatment of Combat Stress

Mary Laedtke

INTRODUCTION

Occupational therapy (OT) has been a part of combat medical support since World War I. The Persian Gulf War provided an opportunity to test the integration of current OT practice in a modern combat environment. The results demonstrated that OT's emphasis on purposeful, useful, productive activity has an important role in staffing and operating combat stress control units.

BACKGROUND

In 1918, military occupational therapists were deployed to Base Hospital No. 117 in France as reconstruction aides in direct treatment of combat stress casualties ("shell shock" in World War I terminology). Purposeful activity and work details were employed by these reconstruction aides. Base Hospital No. 117 returned 50 percent of the shell shock cases to combat duty and 40 percent to other military duty. General Pershing was impressed by these statistics, and he requested the training of additional reconstruction aides. By May 1919, there were over 500 reconstruction aides on active duty in the United States and overseas.

In World War II, civilian occupational therapists were assigned at several echelons of Army hospital care: general, regional, station, and convalescent hospitals. A variety of treatments were provided for neuropsychiatric casualties, amputees, casualties with hand injuries, and casualties with other sensory/motor problems. Lieutenant Colonel Challman, U.S. Army psychiatric consultant to the Southwest Pacific theater of operations, requested the inclusion of occupational therapy in his combat stress treatment program. The success of his program was in part due to the organized day of purposeful work provided by occupational therapists.

U.S. Army occupational therapists and occupational therapy assistants supported operations in the Vietnam War. Starting in 1965, occupational therapists provided third echelon care to soldiers requiring orthotic intervention. Work activities and graded physical activities were provided for soldiers with psychiatric problems, malaria, or hepatitis. In 1971, an occupational therapist spent 10 months as part of Headquarters, U.S. Army Medical Command, Vietnam. The therapist was responsible for developing the occupational therapy components of drug and alcohol treatment programs in Cam Ranh Bay and Long Binh.

From the end of the Vietnam War to the beginning of the Persian Gulf War, the role of occupational therapy in U.S. Army mental health continued to expand. In recent years, occupational therapists have taken part in numerous combat stress field training exercises and have been included in the Army plans for future combat stress control units. On the eve of the Gulf War, a policy decision was made to include occupational therapists in at least one of the corps level mental health teams.

OCCUPATIONAL THERAPY DURING THE GULF WAR

Predeployment

The period between August 15 and September 9, 1990 was one of intense activity in the Office of the Army Surgeon General and U.S. Army Health Services Command in planning the deployment of U.S. Army medical personnel to the Gulf region. As described in the earlier chapter by Holsenbeck (Chapter 4), the 528th Medical Detachment (Psychiatric), a field deployable mental health team, was rapidly constituted and deployed to Saudi Arabia as part of the 18th Airborne Corps.

The formation of the 528th was an opportunity for U.S. Army occupational therapy. Occupational therapists had been involved in numerous recent Army field training exercises, had proved themselves in the field, and were being planned in the formation of the combat stress control teams envisioned in future medical units. However, this concept had not yet been approved or implemented. Thus, occupational therapists were not included in the initial orders forming the 528th. Days and multiple telephone calls later, a decision was made to include an occupational therapist and an occupational therapy technician as replacements for a social worker and a psychiatry technician.

The occupational therapist became part of the 528th treatment team, and the occupational therapy technician joined one of the 528th consultation teams. Their first goal in both teams was the education of team members on occupational therapy's role and the principles of work therapy. The first task was straightforward. The majority of the staff were familiar with the traditional

OT inpatient psychiatry interventions, such as crafts, work therapy, and life skills classes. It was simple for them to adapt work therapy from the inpatient setting to the field environment and to understand the relationship between work therapy and the concept of treating combat stress casualties with brief intervention, near the front, with a plan for rapid return to duty.

Securing OT supplies in preparation for deployment was tedious and frustrating. There were no OT related supplies on the detachment's supply list and no predetermined list for a combat stress occupational therapy section. After action reports from previous field training exercises, lists developed for field-deployable hospitals' occupational therapy packs, and discussions with staff at the Academy of Health Sciences helped identify the required equipment. Standard stock lists for carpenter's toolkits (engineer squad and platoon) were provided by the 36th Engineer Group. Supply requests were submitted, but there was no guarantee of delivery prior to deployment. A personal toolbox with a hammer, screwdrivers, staple gun, vice grips, pliers, etc. was packed as a backup for the equipment on order. Prior to deployment, a limited number of tools did arrive, but the push pack with the majority of the tools never did arrive.

Previous field training exercises had taught the importance of balancing work, play, leisure, and rest, both in treating patients and in the general conduct of operations. Recreational and sport-related equipment, such as volleyballs, footballs, and frisbees, was requested. In addition, several decks of playing cards, a chess set, checkers, and compact travel versions of popular games were chosen. The recreational supplies were procured from a local toy store.

Deployment

The 528th arrived in Saudi Arabia on October 27, 1990. Within a few days, the unit established its first home, a collection of seven tents in the vicinity of Dhahran on the coast in Northeast Saudi Arabia. Although the unit was collocated with a combat support hospital (CSH), the living and treatment areas were established in an area set slightly apart from the CSH. This separation encouraged the idea that participants in the 528th's program were not hospitalized patients but rather soldiers requiring assistance. Soldiers and staff alike lived a spartan existence, sleeping on cots and living in tents. The tents were set up over 50 by 100 foot cement slabs. Sand bags were used to secure the sides of the tents, cover generator cables, and outline sidewalks within the unit's area. A volleyball court was set up. Also set up behind the tents were two four seater latrines. Unit members shared showers and a dining facility with the CSH. Hot meals were provided for breakfast and dinner, while the lunch meal consisted of meals ready to eat (MREs), soup, and fruit.

Each of the six sections comprising the unit (one treatment team and five consultation teams) set up their living area and developed plans for their particular mission. The treatment team worked to set up a living area and designed a treatment program for combat stress casualties. The treatment program was developed cooperatively by the psychiatrist, psychiatric nursing staff, and occupational therapy staff. The program emphasized return to duty, identification of problems that were within the soldier's control, and use of coping mechanisms. It was organized into three phases with the goal of reconstructing from the stress casualty an effective soldier.

Phase I (reconstitution phase) consisted of physical replenishment and restoration. This included a brief respite from duty, food and water, a shower and a change of clothes, and sleep. Psychiatric nursing staff were in charge of this phase.

During phase II (reorientation phase), the program combined education and practical application in work therapy. Soldiers attended educational briefings and participated in work details. Educational briefings included stress management, anger control, assertiveness training, relaxation techniques, and goal setting. Both psychiatric nursing staff and occupational therapy staff facilitated the groups. After attending briefings, soldiers were placed in work therapy assignments throughout our area and in and around the CSH. Occupational therapy was responsible for assigning soldiers to work details. Work therapy provided the occupational therapy personnel an opportunity to evaluate work skills, and gave soldiers a chance to practice the techniques learned in the classes. Each soldier's military occupational specialty was considered in assigning work details. If possible, soldiers were assigned to work details in their area of military occupation. Soldiers who were in combat arms specialties, such as infantryman, tanker, or air defense artillery, were assigned jobs related to their hobbies or general duties necessary for the smooth running of our area and the CSH. In phase III (reintegration) soldiers were required to work the entire day. Soldiers in both phases II and III were also expected to participate in morning and afternoon physical training.

General guidelines for treatment were based on the principles of reconstruction, but more specific detailed decisions had to be made regarding the actual schedule of activities and program rules. Again, the personnel from psychiatry, nursing, and occupational therapy collaborated regarding the daily schedule and acceptable, therapeutic rules. Work activities were scheduled in the morning and late afternoon when it was cooler. Length of work therapy assignments ranged from four to eight hours daily. Classes were held inside the tent during the early afternoon. During classes, soldiers were encouraged to discuss their ability to apply the coping strategies discussed while in their work activity.

Physical activity was scheduled twice a day. The first block of physical training was early in the morning. This physical training was led by the most senior soldier in the program. In the afternoon, everyone played our own unique form of volleyball—affectionately known as "smash mouth" or "combat" volleyball. This was sometimes played in gas masks. It was fun and helped to increase everyone's tolerance for the mask. This physical activity proved to be valuable for both the soldiers in the program and the staff.

The first hurdle for the actual placement of the soldiers in their work details was enlisting the support of the first sergeant of the CSH with which we were collocated. Initially there was reluctance in placing soldiers on work details, as the hospital staff expected the 528th's program to be more like that of traditional inpatient psychiatry. Educating the CSH staff on the difference between an inpatient psychiatry program and combat stress control was a continuing challenge.

Eventually, the first sergeant of the CSH agreed, and a number of work therapy assignments were arranged. The types of assignments included medical supply, communications, unit supply, pharmacy, motor pool, dining facility, field sanitation, personnel, patient administration, laundry, chaplain, and nuclear, biological, and chemical attack protection. Soldiers were also assigned tasks to improve the living environment throughout the area. These included filling sandbags, repairing latrine facilities, disinfecting water bottles, maintaining and repairing volleyball equipment and court, securing tentage, and burying generator cords.

Soldiers in the program were treated as soldiers, not as patients. They were addressed by their military rank, required to be in battle dress uniform, and expected to conduct themselves with proper military bearing. Self responsibility was demanded. Soldiers who chose not to cooperate and were not deemed psychiatrically ill were discharged from the program and, in effect, referred for administrative and/or disciplinary action by their unit.

Upon entering the program, soldiers were interviewed by the psychiatrist, a psychiatric nurse, and an occupational therapist. Each soldier was evaluated daily, and progress (or lack thereof) was discussed at the morning staff meeting. The emphasis was on ability to function as a soldier, not on presence or absence of symptoms.

Our treatment program was in operation from November 3, 1990 to January 9, 1991. During that time, 87 soldiers were enrolled in the program. The average length of stay was three to five days, at which time the soldier was returned to duty with his or her unit. All but eight soldiers were successfully returned to duty.

Soldiers were surprised by the demands, practical focus, and brevity of our program. Many had expected a program more in line with that of an inpatient psychiatry ward. Some lived in better conditions back in their unit than they did when in our stress management program. They did not expect to sleep in a tent on a cot without running water and to use outdoor latrines. They also did not expect that they were going to have to work. The program was not a respite from work, but a working opportunity to apply the stress coping options, if they chose.

Soldier Profiles and the Evaluation of Data

Soldiers completed the Occupational Performance Screening Questionnaire as part of the 528th's combat stress casualty treatment program. The majority of the soldiers were referred because of family problems. Family concerns and difficulty adapting to the demands of deployment (waiting, training, sand, heat, lack of privacy, and uncertainty) appeared to be the main stressors. The most common request was for "two weeks home, just two weeks back home and everything will be okay." Many of the soldiers did not want to be in Saudi Arabia or felt they had been there long enough already. Several soldiers complained that they were tired of the "hurry up and wait" situation and the constant training. While many wanted the war to get started so it could be over, several confessed to being afraid of death or injury.

During December, a decision was made that the three consultation teams, in addition to their work in consultation, would be required to operate as treatment teams for combat stress casualties. The occupational therapy technician was assigned to one of the consultation teams. He began his integration with the consultation team with a one-week stay during December. On January 10, 1991, as the team packed up to move north, the occupational therapy technician became a permanent member of that consultation team.

We had no clear idea of when or where the bulk of the combat stress casualties would turn up, and the treatment team and the consultation teams were constantly repacking and moving, unpacking, repacking and moving again from January 10, 1991 (before the beginning of the air war) through February 28, 1991 (the cease-fire).

There were very few combat stress casualties during the air war or ground war in either the 18th Airborne Corps or the VIIth Corps, the two U.S. Army Corps deployed during the Gulf War. Several reasons have been suggested for such a small number of combat stress casualties. They include the facts that U.S. combat forces were very well prepared. We were victorious, the ground combat was over very quickly, and there were very few American casualties. There were, however, a number of stress related psychiatric cases among the deployed troops in the Gulf region during the lengthy build up period. These deployment casualties offered an opportunity for combat stress control units in the theater of operations to exercise some of their mental health capabilities.

LESSONS LEARNED

Our experience during the Gulf War reinforces the belief that occupational therapy provides a unique contribution to the combat stress team by its emphasis on activities of daily living, purposeful activity, and activity analysis. With the arrival of the 528th Medical Detachment (Psychiatric) in the Gulf theater of operations and its program, which emphasized purposeful activity, rates of evacuation from the theater for psychiatric reasons plummeted.

We learned from our experience that in modern war, the place for combat stress teams is as close to the front as possible. In past field training exercises, occupational therapists were assigned back in the evacuation hospital area. We know now that combat stress casualties need to be treated much closer to the front. Combat stress control teams need to be with the combat support hospitals and mobile Army surgical hospitals in close proximity to the fighting.

The means of returning recovered combat stress casualties to their units is not well organized. Several soldiers were kept longer at the treatment section because their units could not be contacted or because they moved and there was no centralized way of finding out where they had gone. Once units were found, it was difficult to get transportation to return the soldier. The members of the 528th did their best to instill in the soldiers who came to us as a stress casualty the idea that they would soon return to effective duty in their own unit.

Throughout the time that occupational therapy has been involved with combat control teams, the activity provided (work) has always been known as work therapy. The whole point of the combat stress control team is returning a soldier to duty. The term *therapy* construes ill health. Therefore, a healthier, more military description of the occupational therapy component of combat stress control is "work activity or work detail" not "work therapy."

An occupational therapy program cannot be successful without the support and cooperation of the team with which it is working. In the 528th, occupational therapy was fortunate to have a commander who understood the important role of occupational therapy in the treatment of combat stress casualties and believed in its value. The conviction in the value of occupational therapy was shared by the treatment teams' psychiatrists, psychologists, social workers, and other clinical staff.

Logistical support is vital to successful operations. The tools available were limited. The tools requested while in the states never arrived. Tools purchased locally in Saudi Arabia were of poor quality and wore out quickly. OT personnel relied on the few tools that the staff brought with them. There was virtually no wood, so projects had to be made with scrap wood. Packing crates were carefully dismantled so that both the wood and the nails could be used and used again.

Greater numbers of occupational therapy personnel need to be deployed with combat stress control teams. Only two of the four teams had an occupational therapist or technician. With the advent of Medical Force 2000, this problem should be resolved.

The personnel of the 528th had the same opportunities to experience combat stress as the rest of the troops in Saudi Arabia. Unit members had the same potential contributing sources—the stress of mobilization, the stress of an extreme environment, the lack of privacy, the lack of combat experience, the uncertainty about what we would find when we came home, and the distinct likelihood of nuclear, biological, or chemical warfare. Unit members had the same fear of injury or death, the same fear of the unknown as anyone else. But we tried to practice what we preached. We tried to balance work, play, rest, and sleep.

SUMMARY

The Gulf War was an important testing ground for the combat stress control team concept and occupational therapy's role in that team. This experience has demonstrated that there is a role for occupational therapy; the actual work of the combat stress control team cannot be accomplished adequately by the other disciplines alone. Occupational therapists are environmental managers and are the foundation on which the combat stress control teams operate.

Part III

ASSESSING THE GULF WAR EXPERIENCE

14

Unit Cohesion during the Persian Gulf War

Robert K. Gifford, James A. Martin, David H. Marlowe, Kathleen M. Wright, and Paul T. Bartone

INTRODUCTION

As U.S. Army forces deployed to Southwest Asia (the Persian Gulf) to deter Iraqi aggression in the early days of the Gulf War and later prepared to liberate Kuwait, developing and maintaining unit cohesion was a primary concern. The Army Vice Chief of Staff directed the Walter Reed Army Institute of Research (WRAIR) to study coping and adaptation of Army forces in the Persian Gulf, with particular emphasis on unit cohesion. In response to this tasking, the WRAIR deployed a series of small research teams with the initial three-person team arriving in the Persian Gulf in September 1990 and the final team returning from the Persian Gulf in June 1991. These teams interviewed soldiers and administered questionnaires to determine what the key stresses were and how soldiers coped and to assess levels of morale and cohesion. From July through December 1991, military social scientists from the WRAIR conducted follow up interviews and it administered surveys in the United States and Germany to assess postdeployment adaptation.

METHOD

The first team only conducted interviews, having decided before deploying that questionnaire administration would have to be deferred until key issues were better defined and until the theater matured sufficiently to allow transport and distribution of questionnaires. More than 500 deployed soldiers, ranging in rank from private to lieutenant general, took part in these initial semistructured interviews. Interviews were either individual or done with groups of fewer than 10 and were held in soldiers' work or living areas. Those interviewed in groups were always seen with other soldiers of similar rank, without their supervisors being present.   When possible, the interview program included different organizational levels from a given unit.   For example, within a battalion, the commander, command sergeant major, company commanders and first sergeants, platoon leaders, platoon sergeants, squad leaders, and squad members were interviewed in succession.   When operational or time constraints made it impossible to be comprehensive within a unit, enlisted soldiers and junior NCOs were interviewed rather than the senior leaders.

The units visited included maneuver battalions from each of the three divisions then established in the Persian Gulf, as well as support and headquarters units.   The selection of targeted units was done In a manner that ensured that the team saw those units that had been in the Persian Gulf the longest, were the most forward deployed, lived under the most austere conditions, or had missions judged particularly stressful by their higher headquarters.

Interviews normally took between 60 and 90 minutes.   Interviewers had soldiers describe each stage of the deployment from the time they were notified through the time of the interview.   The major stressors at each stage were discussed, and soldiers were asked what individual coping mechanisms, unit supports, or leader actions helped them cope with these stressors.   The interviews were open ended, and soldiers were encouraged to bring up issues they saw as most important, both in describing stress points and in evaluating coping and adaptation techniques.

The information from these interviews was incorporated in a plan for studying the maturing theater, which included questionnaires as well as additional interviewing.   To accomplish this plan, a second research team returned to the Persian Gulf theater in November 1990 and interviewed over 800 soldiers (using the same basic format described earlier) and administered questionnaires to 1200 soldiers from eight combat arms battalions (two each from the four divisions then in the Persian Gulf).

The questionnaire took about 45 minutes to complete and was administered at unit field sites.   The questionnaire included demographic questions, items measuring the soldiers' beliefs about Army family support, measures of unit cohesion (both vertical cohesion up and down the chain of command, and horizontal cohesion among peers), perceptions of leader effectiveness, sections in which soldiers rated the stressfulness of various aspects of the deployment and the effectiveness of different coping techniques, and the Brief Symptom Inventory, a measure of psychological distress (Derogatis and Spencer, 1982). Sometimes surveys were given to soldiers directly by the research team, while on other occasions, surveys were distributed and collected by the chain of command.   Although it is not possible to calculate response rates, given the necessity of opportunity sampling and the need to be flexible in method of distribution, the researchers' impression was that most soldiers who were actually given the questionnaire filled it out.   Nonresponders seem to have been primarily those whose duties precluded their receiving the survey. There is no reason to believe that the sample was not representative of the units surveyed.

In January 1991 (after the start of the air war), a shortened version of the questionnaire was administered in a VIIth Corps division and an armored cavalry regiment.   The abbreviated version included both unit cohesion measures and shortened symptom inventory, but it omitted the sections dealing with deployment stressors and focused instead on stress relating to anticipation of combat.

Postcombat surveying began in May 1991, with soldiers still in the Persian Gulf, and continued with follow-up visits to units redeployed to their home posts in the United States and Germany.   Surveying continued through November 1991.   Approximately 9200 usable surveys were obtained in this wave of data collection.   The postcombat surveys included the cohesion measures and the Brief Symptom Inventory as used in the precombat surveys, as well as the Impact of Events Scale (Horowitz, Wilner, and Alvarez, 1979), a hardiness scale to measure individual psychological resilience (Bartone et al., 1989), a scale assessing exposure to combat and the soldiers' ratings of the stress of this exposure, and a number of items relating to homecoming and reunion issues.

RESULTS AND DISCUSSION

On the basis of their initial interviews in September–October 1990, the first research team concluded that individual morale was good and small unit cohesion was at a high level. Soldiers were enduring the uncertain situation and difficult living conditions well. This is not to say that they did not find these conditions stressful. On the contrary, most soldiers had complaints about a variety of issues related to the deployment. Further questioning usually revealed that they were functioning extraordinarily well given the circumstances under which they were operating and in spite of their frustration with primitive living conditions and the pain of separation from family and friends.

Problems for units in either morale or cohesion could generally be traced to factors that existed before the deployment. Units in which there were deficiencies in trust or communication up and down the chain of command prior to the Gulf War in most cases did not improve as a result of deployment. On the contrary, during the first months of the Gulf War, the stresses and intense interpersonal contact incident to deployment often exacerbated problems that had existed at the unit's home station in the United States. Similarly, soldiers' individual problems that existed before the alert often continued or became worse after deployment. While such instances of isolated low individual morale or weak unit cohesion were distressing to the soldiers involved, they do not detract from the more important observation that the majority of military units and individual soldiers were coping well in a highly stressful and demanding environment.

These subjective conclusions, by interviewers experienced in studying cohesion in military units, received quantitative support from the questionnaires administered in December 1990. Of the 25 companies from XVIIIth Airborne Corps that took the survey, 23 had mean vertical cohesion scores higher than the mean score for the same scale in WRAIR studies conducted from 1985 through 1989, and 24 of 25 were higher on the horizontal cohesion scale. In a situation as intense and rapidly changing as the Gulf War deployment, there can never be precise, well controlled measurement of variables such as cohesion. The survey data strongly support the notion that unit cohesion was indeed high during the early deployment.

The interviews conducted in November–December 1990 supported the earlier findings and further showed how maturation of the theater was affecting morale and cohesion. Increased availability of various amenities in the theater (e.g., more showers, better tents, better food, occasional cold soft drinks) helped compensate for the austerity of life in the Persian Gulf, and, perhaps more importantly, demonstrated to soldiers that the chain of command did care about them.

The announcement by the Secretary of Defense that U.S. forces would not rotate out of the theater but would stay until the issue of Kuwait was resolved also affected morale. Although many soldiers were at first disappointed not to be given a date to return home, the ultimate effect of this decision was morale enhancing, as soldiers now had a clear mission and, if not a date for return, at least a statement of what events must occur before they could go home. The January 15 deadline set by the United Nations further clarified the situation and allowed soldiers to focus their thinking on the nature of the task ahead.

A number of factors undoubtedly led to the generally high levels of cohesion observed by the interview teams and confirmed by the questionnaire results. In interviews, both soldiers and their leaders cited the time they spent living and training in the desert as the key factor in developing cohesion. A sense of shared purpose caused them to learn to take care of each other, initially in order to survive in the desert during the early phase of the deployment, and then to prepare for war.

While the crowding and close living quarters prevalent in the theater were stressful, these conditions also forced unit members to develop skills in living with each other and resolving interpersonal problems, since there was no opportunity to get away from the unit. The "for the duration" announcement and the January 15 deadline gave the soldiers a sense of purpose, as well as a clear realization of their interdependence. The exceptional personnel stability achieved by combat arms units deployed to the Persian Gulf also contributed to cohesion. Because transfers out of units were minimal during the Gulf War, there was a relatively long period in which the same soldiers could work and train together at the squad and crew levels. Some leaders noted in interviews that the levels of stability achieved and the training opportunities this stability provided were similar to what was envisioned by the Army when the COHORT (acronym for Cohesion, Operational Readiness, and Training) unit manning system was developed in the early 1980s (Marlowe, 1987)

There were, of course, differences among units in levels of cohesion. Leader behavior and family support emerged from interviews and questionnaire data as key determinants of cohesion. Leaders who provided information, showed personal interest in the welfare of their soldiers, and shared burdens with them obtained higher levels of cohesion in their units. These sets of behaviors interacted; for example, one way for leaders to show their interest in the welfare of soldiers was to ensure that information—including news as well as operational plans—was passed to soldiers. Soldiers, when asked what made them believe their leaders cared for them, often cited the fact that their chain of command did what it could to keep them informed. Similarly, leaders who shared burdens with soldiers, such as austere living conditions or physically demanding tasks, were seen as interested in the welfare of their soldiers. Actions taken by leaders to provide basic amenities for soldiers acquired an important symbolic value, as facilities such as showers or better tents represented, in the eyes of the soldiers, the willingness of their leaders to support them.

Soldiers in the most cohesive units also reported more confidence that the family support systems at their home posts would care for their families if needed. The correlation's between both vertical and horizontal cohesion scores and responses to five survey questions rating confidence in family support were all statistically significant and substantial (Pearson r values ranged from .23 to 42, all p-values < .01) in the sample of 1200 XVIIIth Airborne Corps soldiers surveyed in December 1990. The Army has long held that family support is a component of readiness. In view of these correlations, the Gulf War experience supports this view.

The consequences of the high levels of cohesion observed during the deployment and build-up phases of the Gulf War were evident in the postcombat interview and questionnaire results. Soldiers and leaders alike stated that the opportunity to build cohesion while training in the desert was a key factor in their ability to accomplish their mission effectively and with so few casualties when the ground war came. Further, cohesion was positively correlated with postcombat adjustment and health indicators. The more cohesive the unit, the fewer symptoms its members reported on the Impact of Events Scale and the Brief Symptoms Inventory in the postcombat surveys (Bartone et al., 1992).

SUMMARY

The present research supports the thesis that unit cohesion contributes to combat success and to postcombat adjustment. The data from the Gulf War need further analysis to delineate the precise mechanisms by which high levels of cohesion were created and how the beneficial effects of cohesion can be maximized. The other key questions are whether units were able to maintain the high levels of cohesion achieved in the desert after their return from the Gulf War and whether the positive effects on health and adjustment continue over time.

REFERENCES

Bartone, P.T., R.K. Gifford, K.M. Wright, D.H. Marlowe, and J.A. Martin. (1992, June). *U.S. Soldiers Remain Healthy Under Gulf War Stress*. Paper presented at the 4th Annual Convention of the American Psychological Society, San Diego, Calif.

Bartone, P. T., R. J. Ursano, K. M. Wright, and L. H. Ingraham. (1989). "The impact of a military air disaster on the health of assistance workers." *J. Nerv. Mental Dis.*, 177(6): 317–328.

Derogatis, L. R. and P M. Spencer. (1982). *The Brief Symptom Inventory (BSI): Administration, Scoring, And Procedures Manual — I.* Baltimore: Johns Hopkins.

Horowitz, M., N. Wilner, and W. Alvarez. (1979). "Impact of Events Scale: A measure of subjective stress." *Psychosomatic Med.* 41(3):209–218.

Marlowe, D. H. (ed.) (1987). *New Manning System Field Evaluation: Technical Report No. 5.* Washington, D.C.: Walter Reed Army Institute of Research.

15

Mental Health Lessons from the Persian Gulf War

James A. Martin and William R. Cline

INTRODUCTION

This chapter documents important mental health issues from the Gulf War. It is based on presentations and discussions at a combined Combat Psychiatry Training Course/"Operation Desert Shield/Storm (ODS) Lessons Learned" Conference held at Vilseck, Germany, October 6 through October 9, 1991. Conference participants included U.S. Army mental health officers who served in the Gulf War or provided mental health services in the United States and/or Europe during this period, along with the senior British Army psychiatrist in the Gulf War and the senior U.S. Navy psychiatrist from the *U.S.S. Comfort* (one of the Navy hospital ships deployed during the Gulf War).

The mental health lessons learned highlighted here focus on structural and operational problems observed during the Gulf War. The list is long. Despite these concerns, there are a number of mental health success stories that need to be mentioned first.

SOME SUCCESSFUL EFFORTS

During the predeployment phase, a number of division and military community mental health professionals provided unit leaders and soldiers with valuable didactic information on a variety of operational stress issues. Often, classes on combat stress were built right into unit-level predeployment orientations.

Family issues received enormous attention. Mental health officers (along with other community caregivers) provided soldiers and their families with guidance on a variety of stress and coping issues. In many communities, this help extended into the school system and included efforts to support the emotional needs of the children of deploying soldiers. An extensive network of unit and community support provided soldiers with considerable reassurance that their families would be well cared for during their absence.

Early into the deployment of forces to Saudi Arabia, the Army theater surgeon added a psychiatric consultant to his staff. This was based on his recognition of the importance of mental health issues in sustaining a force in this physically, psychologically, and socially stressful theater of operations, and it underscored the critical concern about battle fatigue as a potential source of combat medical casualties. Unfortunately, a qualified consultant did not arrive until December 1990, too late to influence the mental health issues associated with the build up phase. The presence of the psychiatry consultant in the theater did occur in time for necessary shifting and restructuring of mental health resources in preparation for the ground offensive. The consultant also created a mental health safety net that conference participants believed would have effectively prevented any hemorrhaging of mental health casualties from this theater had the originally predicted level of combat causalities occurred.

During the highly stressful prewar period, a number of corps and division mental health officers and behavioral science specialist demonstrated the effectiveness of aggressive command consultation and brief, highly focused mental health interventions. In these forward deployed units, very few soldiers required evacuation. Brief rest (often only a few hours of sleep) usually provided a powerful restorative effect. Treatment interventions helped soldiers to focus on issues within their immediate control and were usually enough to restore soldiers to effective duty.

A few division mental health teams demonstrated that it is possible to provide care forward even in fast-moving ground operations. The mental health team formed to support one of the armored cavalry regiments demonstrated the capability and value of systematic after action debriefings for traumatized combat teams still in forward positions.

Finally, the Gulf War provided a generation of active and reserve mental health officers with wartime skills. Their experience and knowledge needs to be captured and integrated into our training and doctrine. The following critical issues and recommendations, which emerged from their lessons learned conference discussions, provide a starting point. These lessons center around clinical, personnel, and structural concerns.

Clinical issues include training for combat mental health readiness, management of psychiatric casualties, combat stress control restoration in airland battle operations, support for return to duty of battle fatigue casualties, development of operational plans (referred to as OPLANs) for psychiatry services, and small unit after-action stress debriefings.

Personnel issues include the need for a theater-level neuropsychiatry consultant, the need for a corps psychiatry staff officer, problems with the

Professional Officer Filler System (PROFIS), and the need to correct problems associated with the assignment of behavioral science specialists.

Structural issues include mental health support for brigade or larger independent units, division mental health sections, location of corps-level mental health units/personnel, medical detachment psychiatric (OM) team deficiencies, the need for mental health support for all combat theater hospitals, and combat stress control and joint/combined operations.

ISSUES AND RECOMMENDATIONS

Clinical Issues

Training for Combat Mental Health Readiness. Most mental health officers have some theoretical training in the prevention and treatment of combat stress reactions—what will be referred to in this chapter by the term used in current Army doctrine, *battle fatigue.* Unfortunately, at the time of the Gulf War, many mental health officers and enlisted personnel lacked hands-on experience operating in unit/field environments, and they lacked basic soldier skills necessary for effective functioning in a combat environment. A number of inexperienced and poorly prepared mental health officers and enlisted soldiers were deployed to the Gulf War. Had they not had several months in the combat theater to prepare themselves, they would have poorly served soldiers who suffered from battle fatigue and may well have become causalities themselves.

To minimize these problems, Army mental health officers and enlisted personnel should not be assigned to divisions (or to corps level combat stress control companies [CSCCs] and combat stress control detachments [CSCDs]) as a first assignment after completing their clinical training. Many could serve well after a first assignment in a hospital setting, and mental health officers with training obligations should expect their second assignment to be in a division mental health team or to a CSCC or CSCD. Combat stress control training must be built into division training schedules. CSCCs and CSCDs must also train in field environments on a regular basis.

A multidisciplined combat mental health training conference for active and reserve component officers and senior enlisted personnel should be conducted annually to review combat mental health principles and practice skills. This training should take place at a combat arms Army training center where real-world combat training activities can be integrated into the conference.

Management of Psychiatric Casualties. Both Operation Just Cause in Panama and the Gulf War demonstrate that combat leaders and senior medical officers assume, and initially desire, immediate evacuation of all casualties out of the theater of operations. They are not focused on returning the soldier to fight in the next battle. The line commander wants to get the injured soldier to the best possible medical care and to get him or her out of the way of any additional danger. The line commander is focused on a quick, decisive battle, starting with sufficient forces so that replacements are not an issue. This means deploying only a limited medical presence in order to maximize the delivery of combat forces and equipment into the combat theater.

Senior medical officers are focused on surgical wound casualties, whose potential arrival in large numbers requires keeping the hospital census low. Except for "lightly injured or minor illness" (especially when there is an avoidance aspect to the condition), most medical and surgical evacuations out of the theater are medically beneficial or at least not psychologically harmful (although these soldiers often require mental health support to cope with the stress associated with their medical conditions).

For the battle-fatigued soldier, evacuation is a treatment approach that goes against medical doctrine and creates the risk of subsequent serious social and psychiatric complications. Avoidable posttraumatic stress syndrome is the most likely consequence. Thus, when viewed objectively, inappropriate evacuation may constitute medical malpractice.

While one of the goals of returning battle-fatigued soldiers to their unit is to provide replacement soldiers, the other goal is to support the soldier's psychological recovery, including the prevention of subsequent psychiatric disability. Returning a recovered battle-fatigued soldier to his or her own unit (and peer group) is the treatment of choice. This is true even if the soldier can not be returned until after the battle is over (or returned during a break in fighting when the unit is being resupplied).

The worst mental health outcomes follow inappropriate evacuation out of the combat theater; soldiers can be lost to military service or effective civilian functioning. Returning the battle fatigued soldier to the original unit is usually therapeutic. The battle-fatigued soldier will have a personal set of war stories to tell and will have the opportunity to reintegrate into the small group. The battle-fatigued soldier evacuated out of the theater will never have this opportunity and is at greater risk for permanent psychological and social dysfunction.

Conference participants concluded that there needs to be a clear distinction made in applying evacuation policies (and practices) to battle-fatigued soldiers versus other casualties so that all leaders (including medical officers) understand that the best possible treatment occurs in the theater of operations. The focus must be returning the soldier to duty in the original unit while the unit is still in theater. Mental health resources must exist at all theater level evacuation sites to ensure that battle-fatigued soldiers are not prematurely evacuated out of theater.

Commanders and senior medical officers need to be better informed about the proper treatment of battle fatigue and the clinical importance of returning soldiers to their original unit as soon as possible. There is also a need to build combat stress control holding into operations orders, as well as peacetime training simulations and field training exercises.

Combat Stress Control Restoration—AirLand Battle Operations. In the Gulf War, brigades operated with the high mobility and pace called for in the Army's doctrine called AirLand Battle Operations. With this speed and resulting great operational distances, division main support elements were often left far behind their division's combat units. In any conflict that involves a series of battles, soldiers evacuated behind the brigades would have no chance of returning within the one to two days suggested by doctrine. Corps level mental health teams (designated as OM teams) were too few, too untrained in combat survival skills, and had too few reliable vehicles to reinforce forward support medical companies (as called for in doctrine). Had there been prolonged fighting and/or high numbers of wounded and corresponding stress casualties, most divisions would not have had even minimally sufficient forward holding capabilities.

To alleviate these problems, the Army needs to continue fielding combat stress control (CSC) companies and detachments and sustain these units with an enhanced tables of organization and equipment (TO&Es) that will improve the number, tactical mobility, and carrying capacity of their vehicles. These mental health teams need a tactical ambulance to provide evaluation and quick treatment while on the move. CSC restoration team need additional mobile holding capability (for example, a 5 ton truck with tents and ground pads or cots, plus restoration-specific gear). Combat stress control holding capability should be in the brigade support areas or as close behind the brigades as is feasible in the medical task force. There is a need to continue to refine Army Medical Department (AMEDD) combat stress control doctrine focused on far forward treatment in environments that will always require the kind of flexibility and improvisation only possible in well trained units.

U.S. Army Adjutant General (Personnel) Support for Return to Duty of Battle Fatigue Casualties. The Gulf War demonstrated that once a soldier reaches a nonorganic medical treatment facility (e.g., a rearward combat support hospital or an evacuation hospital) and the soldier's brigade has moved forward, the personnel system provides no way to move the soldier from the medical treatment facility back to the unit.

Return to the original unit as soon as possible is critical in psychological recovery as well as important in reducing the likelihood of subsequent psychiatric dysfunction and permanent disability. It reinforces for other soldiers that battle fatigue does not provide a quick, easy way home. Any delay in returning a recovered battle-fatigued soldier to duty decreases the likelihood of successful reintegration and increases the chances of continued dysfunction and future psychiatric disability. For soldiers unsuitable for return to their unit (for any of a variety of reasons), other assignments in the theater are needed.

The medical and the personnel community must find a way to support the requirement of returning battle-fatigued soldiers to their forward deployed units.

This is an issue that involves doctrine, organization, training, and the requirement to find a way to insert recovered battle-fatigued soldiers into the forward moving replacement/resupply system so that they reach their original units in a timely manner.

Development of Operational Plans (OPLANs) for Psychiatry Services. United States Army Europe (USAREUR) medical facilities were designated the initial out of theater evacuation location for soldiers evacuated from the Gulf War. Prior to the start of the Gulf War, there was no OPLAN at Headquarters, 7th Medical Command in Germany (HQ 7th MEDCOM) for managing battle fatigue casualties evacuated from the Gulf War to USAREUR hospitals (USAREUR hospitals were designated as the primary evacuation sites). In late November 1990, an OPLAN psychiatric annex was published. Despite this plan and guidance from the psychiatry consultant, designated 7th MEDCOM hospitals never developed doctrinally based facilities or treatment programs for managing evacuated battle fatigue casualties. These facilities did adequately manage the routine (noncombat) psychiatric evacuations from the Gulf War. Figure 15.1 highlights the fact that psychiatric casualties represented 6.5 percent of all patients evacuated through USAREUR during the one-year period of the Gulf War, and Figure 15.2 suggests that the percentages of psychiatric casualties evacuated to Europe decreased as mental health resources increased in the theater of operations. This was true until after the ground war ended. At that point, the evacuation percentage increased again, consistent with the fact that mental health personnel were caught up in the emotional desire to redeploy back to the United States and they were not focused on postcombat mental health requirements. It is important to note that almost all evacuated military personnel were sent back to the United States (or their community in U.S. Army Europe). Very few of these soldiers returned to their unit in Southwest Asia.

For these reasons, a current psychiatry annex is needed in all headquarters OPLANs Armywide. Implementing a change from peacetime psychiatric care to care for battle fatigue casualties requires a major program change with operational guidance from a military psychiatrist with specific battle fatigue management training and/or combat experience. There seems to be significant advantages to setting up one theater-level battle fatigue restoration center adjacent to a hospital. This center should give soldiers the impression of being in a garrison type environment, instead of a hospital.

All hospitals receiving medical and surgical casualties have a requirement for consultation/liaison psychiatry to evaluate and support physically injured and ill soldiers who have social and psychological problems. Such soldiers, when physical problems are resolved, should be considered for placement in the restoration center if their psychological status is such that effective return to duty is inhibited.

Figure 15.1
Gulf War Patients Evacuated to USAREUR Medical Facilities
2 August 90 to 15 July 91

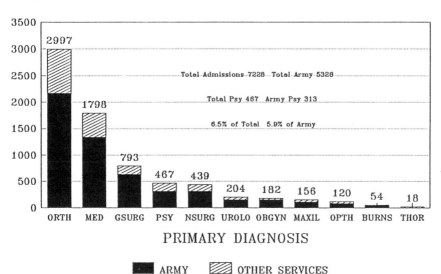

Figure 15.2
Gulf War Psychiatric Casualties Evacuated to 7th MEDCOM
Psychiatric Casualties as a Percent of all Evacuations:
2 August 90 to 15 July 91

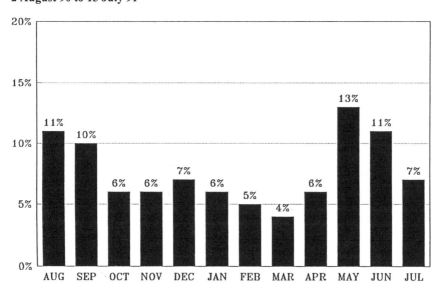

Small Unit After Action Stress Debriefings. After action stress debriefings (similar to what the civilian literature refers to as critical incident stress debriefings) are a recognized method of providing first aid and/or a preventive inoculation to individuals who have been exposed to extreme trauma.   Their success reduces later incidence of posttraumatic stress disorder. Debriefings are considered important in preventing battle fatigue and subsequent posttraumatic stress disorder.

Even in a war that was extremely successful, very brief, and with few American casualties, there were recognizable pockets of trauma. There were soldiers who witnessed the horrors associated with dismemberment and death (whether friend or foe); soldiers who experienced the terror and pain of friendly fire (whether inflicting or receiving); soldiers confronted with the task of handling dismembered and decaying human remains; and soldiers who encountered first hand the pain and suffering of the men, women, and especially the children made refugees by war.

Unfortunately, debriefings were not consistently performed during the post–Gulf War period. Some mental health personnel/units did not recognize this as part of their mission, and others were not adequately trained to perform this service.   The situation was worsened by the general lack of mental health consultation to commanders before combat.   The lack of peacetime mental health command consultation to unit commanders also meant that unit leaders were not always receptive to this support. Where debriefings were performed, soldiers were very appreciative and there were often noticeable positive changes in individual and small group behaviors and attitudes.

After action stress debriefings should become a standard operational procedure whenever a small unit (or group of soldiers) experiences extreme stress (whether in garrison, training, peacetime operations, or combat). Officer and NCO leaders need to be informed about the debriefing process during their leadership development training.   These combat stress debriefings should be incorporated into all field training exercises. This is not a foreign concept for line officers and NCOs, who are already familiar with the notion of after action operational reviews as standard procedure at the National Training Center and other unit training sites.

During the Gulf War, medical leaders were often the most resistant to these services, and they need this same leader orientation. All mental health care providers (including enlisted specialists) need to be trained to conduct these debriefings. The Army surgeon general (in conjunction with the other Service surgeons general and appropriate civilian institutions) should also sponsor additional research on this topic.

Mental Health Personnel Issues

Need for a Theater-Level Neuropsychiatry Consultant.   A mental health consultant was requested by the Army Central Command (ARCENT) Surgeon in October 1990. Unfortunately, a qualified consultant did not arrive in the Gulf until mid December. This lack of senior staff consultation was one of many factors that led to delayed and insufficient deployment of mental health resources into the Gulf War theater of operations.

A mental health consultant should be a designated member of all senior Army level staffs (Surgeon's staff) and involved from the start in contingency planning. The neuropsychiatry consultant should be among the first members of the headquarters staff (in the position of staff surgeon) to deploy into the theater of operations (ideally, this should occur before the deployment of mental health units).

Need for a Corps Psychiatry Staff Officer.   Realizing that the deployed 7th Corps for Germany would have a size far greater than a usual corps and that the worst case scenario anticipated large numbers of psychiatric casualties, the 7th Corps surgeon requested and was provided a staff psychiatrist for the Gulf War deployment. Because of the way the Corps Medical Brigade was organized and operated as a subordinate element of the Corps Support Command, it was not possible to fully test the concept of a corps psychiatry staff officer.

This issue needs further evaluation. Given the array of mental health/human service issues and programs operating during peacetime with very limited senior-level technical supervision, there may also be a valuable role for a corps psychiatry staff officer as a member of the corps surgeon's peacetime staff. One possibility would be to make the medical brigade staff psychiatrist's peacetime position that of the corps psychiatry staff officer.

PROFIS Deficiencies.   Many active duty (and reserve) PROFIS fillers to corps and division mental health team were inadequately trained and prepared for any type of deployment. The Army Reserve Personnel System also failed to fill the reserve OM detachment psychiatry vacancies (although it had a good pool of qualified mental health officers). Two reserve psychiatrists, whose poor physical conditions and ages (58 and 63) and lack of military experience and training made them unsuitable for OM team duties, were sent to the Gulf War theater. Some of the clinical positions on the reserve OM team (especially social work officer and enlisted mental health positions) were filled by individuals who lacked appropriate clinical credentials and had not practiced in their respective fields for many years. A lack of current clinical skills was also an issue for some active duty members whose pre–Gulf War assignments were nonclinical in nature.

The conference participants recommended giving PROFIS assignments to the best qualified personnel to alleviate these deficiencies. Regular field training/unit interface should be provided for all PROFIS personnel. Mental health officers and enlisted members must be required to obtain and maintain necessary clinical skills/credentials.

Behavioral Science Specialist (91G) Authorized Rank and Assignment Policy. The 1984–1985 Medical System Program Review explicitly promised the Army Vice Chief of Staff (General Thurman) a Sergeant First Class Behavior Science Specialist (SFC91G) dedicated to each maneuver brigade. Two efforts to change the Standards of Grade Authorizations failed for lack of a "billpayer" (in a zero sum personnel environment, it required modifying another enlisted specialty to provide these positions—none were identified to pay this personnel bill). One armored division (among others) deployed to the Gulf War with two soldiers just out of advanced individual training (AIT). Their deployment in this role was unfair to the individuals and to the division mental health team. Rather than being an asset, they burdened the division mental health staff. At the time of the division's deployment, there were a number of local senior 91Gs (local hospital assets) volunteering to replace these new soldiers, but substitutions were not allowed. Across the deployed division mental health team, there was almost universal agreement that 91G sergeants and below were not able to function independently at forward support medical companies because they either lacked necessary experience and/or maturity as well as organizational credibility.

Army regulations (AR 611-201) should be amended to specify a behavioral science specialist sergeant first class, one per maneuver brigade, as the brigade combat stress control coordinator. This should be done whether or not the 91G career field is reformed. The combat arms are entitled to their full share of senior 91Gs.

Structural Issues

Mental Health Support for Brigade-Sized or Larger Independent Units. Independent brigades or units, like armored cavalry regiments, do not have organic mental health support. Mental health personnel need time with a unit in order to assess unit needs, develop relationships with leaders that will permit effective command consultation, and, in general, gain an operational familiarity with the people and methods of operation. This did not occur in the Gulf War. By chance rather than design, two brigade (plus)-sized units did receive mental health team just before the start of the ground war. These team were able to provide valuable debriefings for unit personnel exposed to trauma like friendly fire and other accidental deaths and severe injuries.

Other independent (or attached) brigade sized-task forces also lacked mental health support. A review of issues like friendly fire deaths and injuries and other significant psychological trauma suggests that these independent units experienced a large number of these events. At least one of these units did not have mental health support readily available for their soldiers before, during, or subsequent to these events, and there are anecdotal data indicating considerable postcombat distress among soldiers in this unit.

No brigade-sized task force (or armored cavalry regiment) should deploy for any type of operational mission without mental health personnel as part of their organic medical support. These units should be provided with mental health personnel well in advance of any deployment (an ideal augmentation would include at least one mental health officer and two senior 91Gs). Mental health personnel likely to deploy in these units should train with the same unit on a regular basis.

Effectiveness of Division Mental Health Sections. With a few notable exceptions, division mental health team were not effective in providing consultation to commanders or direct psychiatric services to soldiers. Many division mental health officers and enlisted personnel were too junior (in grade and experience) to elicit the respect and confidence of mid-to senior-level commanders, and they often lacked basic soldier skills. Military experience (including the ability to identify with the line) may be even more critical than rank as a factor in success.

At the time of deployment notification, many of the division mental health team lacked critical officer and enlisted personnel. In the two divisions that deployed from Germany, four of six officers and a corresponding number of enlisted specialists were designated at the last minute because positions were vacant or individuals were nondeployable. Overall, five of the seven Army divisions deployed without their full complement of personnel in spite of the fact that qualified soldiers were available in their respective military communities. Cross leveling guidance often prevented team from filling enlisted vacancies with the best readily available personnel, and frequently team were required to deploy with filler personnel who were not adequately trained and/or qualified for their position.

In garrison, requirements to deliver peacetime mental health care directly interfere with training for combat and with command consultation activities (including educating leaders on the use and value of these services). Mental health officers and enlisted personnel rarely participate in significant field training exercises, such as those at the Army's National Training Center in California or any of USAREUR's 7th Army Training Center locations. In garrison, most division mental health team do not have or do not know the location of important equipment, such as vehicles and communication equipment.

Division mental health team deployed to the Gulf War were not adequately staffed to serve their greatly expanded (task organized) divisions. Many divisions were deployed and/or task organized 30 percent to 40 percent larger than their peacetime operational size. Because OM team were not in theater in adequate quantity, there was no way to augment the mental health team in our vastly oversized deployed divisions.

At a minimum, a division mental health team should have one officer and one senior NCO per deployed brigade task force. Based on Gulf War experiences with the 2nd Armored Cavalry Regiment and "Tiger Brigade" of the 2nd Armored Division, these expanded brigade task forces appear to be ideally suited for the assignment and/or attachment of a two-to four-person mental health team. In both cases cited, the presence of mental health personnel during and immediately after combat allowed for the provision of useful debriefings among small units/sections involved in traumatic events like friendly fire. The United Kingdom psychiatric consultant deployed to the Gulf War theater has also recommended assigning and operating mental health sections at brigade level. This is a practice already implemented in the Israeli Defense Forces.

It is suggested that division mental health officers should be AMEDD Advanced Course graduates in the rank of (or selected for) major. The division psychiatrist should not be assigned to the division as a first assignment after residency training. During advanced course training (or as a temporary duty upon selection for a division assignment), division mental health officers should receive a special orientation/practice course on the prevention and management of battle fatigue at division and corps levels. This training should include the topic of after action stress debriefings.

Division mental health enlisted positions should begin at the rank of sergeant (the ideal is a sergeant first class who can operate as a brigade level combat stress control officer). The criterion for filling positions in any deploying division mental health team should be the best qualified individual, and filling from local medical treatment facilities should be allowed. This is especially critical for filling enlisted positions.

Division mental health team need to make clinical care their secondary peacetime activity; the local medical treatment facility should have primary responsibility for ongoing peacetime clinical care requirements, including administrative and medical board actions. Division mental health team activities should focus primarily on command consultation and combat stress prevention and training.

An element of the division mental health section should participate in every major division field training exercise. This will require making "combat stress play" a part of the overall command training plan. This training should be reinforced and evaluated by assigning a mental health officer (or senior 91G) to the evaluation staff at all major combat training centers. No battalion or brigade-sized task force should operationally deploy without taking an element of the division mental health team as a part of its organic medical support.

Upon deployment to a combat zone, sufficient division mental health resources should be available to assign one officer and one NCO to each combat brigade task force. In a combat zone, limited battle fatigue holding capacity should exist within every division main support area.

Location of Corps-Level Mental Health Units/Personnel. The mental health units deployed during the Gulf War were usually available to locate at local medical treatment facilities. During the prolonged pre and post combat period, this made it very difficult for units without organic mental health resources to find adequate mental health care for their soldiers. Medical treatment facilities are typically located with ease of access in mind, but many military medical facilities in the Gulf War theater lacked mental health capabilities. Conference participants estimated that fully 20 percent of the soldiers returned from the Gulf through USAREUR hospitals for psychiatric reasons (August 1, 1990 through August 1, 1991) were evacuated by nonpsychiatric medical staff. This figure does not include a potentially significant number of additional medical and surgical patients who should have been screened and/or cared for by a mental health officer prior to recommending and/or effecting evacuation (there are indications that a substantial number of these evacuated soldiers had medical conditions exacerbated by home front stressors).

In any intense and prolonged combat with significant numbers of stress casualties, locating and evacuating soldiers to mental health treatment units would be difficult unless the mental health unit was located in the vicinity of an identifiable medical treatment facility.

Finally, mental health units are austerely staffed and equipped. These units are not self sufficient and require external sustainment (food, water, resupply, vehicle repair, etc.), especially during periods when they are managing a significant patient population. This is an added rationale for collocating mental health units with medical treatment facilities (at division, corps, and theater levels).

Medical Detachment Psychiatric (OM) Team Deficiencies. The OM team TO&E was known to be obsolete and deficient in mobility and patient holding capability. Combat stress control companies and combat stress control detachments (CSCCs and CSCDs) were in the final stage of Army approval (what had been a very lengthy 16 month bureaucratic process), but the OM team were not allowed to upgrade to the proposed CSCC standard. Only three OM team were deployed (all at "C3-minus" or less than fully capable status), and they either never received their full fill of personnel or, if they did, these personnel did not arrive in a timely manner. These three team represented only 40 percent of the minimum basis of allocation by recognized planning standards. With their deficiencies in required equipment, they represented about 25 percent of the minimum combat deployment requirement.

While the execution of a combat deployment may require limiting mental health personnel/units to a number below the recognized planning standard, mental health resources available during the Gulf War were grossly deficient. Deployed OM team were not adequately staffed, equipped, or trained. Had we faced the worst case scenario for surgical casualties, the medical evacuation system might have been severely stressed by inappropriate psychiatric evacuations.   Even with the best case scenario which occurred, a direct consequence of the late deployment of OM team was excessive evacuation of soldiers with minor psychiatric problems and psychosomatic conditions during the early phase of the Gulf War.

During contingency operations, mental health team should be deployed early and in quantity indicated by current doctrine. Without such full deployment, large independent units (such as the armored cavalry regiments) are at special risk of being without mental health support. Well before deployment, clear identification of personnel should take place, and units should train together. In divisions, at least one mental health officer and NCO should deploy as part of the initial medical contingent. The same principle applies for deployment of corps and theater medical assets.

Adequate mental health resources must be maintained in the theater until force withdrawal is complete, allowing time for postoperations and combat debriefings and reunion/homecoming counseling. Mental health care provided to soldiers experiencing the severe stress associated with refugee care (like support to Kurdish refugees during Operation Provide Comfort) demonstrates the importance of deploying CSCCs and CSCDs to humanitarian military missions.

Need for Mental Health Support for All Combat Theater Hospitals. All field hospitals received stress casualties during the Gulf War. Some hospitals had significant numbers of psychiatric patients in their holding wards. Overevacuation of precombat psychiatric patients and later stress casualties occurred by way of these hospitals, especially in the period before the arrival of the first OM team into the theater of operations. It occurred again when OM team moved forward in preparation for the start of the ground war. Every field hospital provided primary care to units in their area. Mental health services need to be a part of primary care.

All combat support field and general hospitals should have mental health assets. The MASH (Mobile Army Surgical Hospital) should be allocated one psychiatric nurse (66C), who can also function as a surgical nurse. This solution has been adopted by the Navy in their surgical team reinforcing amphibious landing ships (serving as emergency surgical centers).

Combat Stress Control in Joint/Combined Operations. U.S. Air Force mental health personnel deployed early with air transportable hospitals, but they were not located or trained to support Army combat stress control needs. Navy hospital ships are not suitable for Army combat stress control return-to-duty requirements due to inherent hospital environment and return transportation problems. Navy doctrine and training for combat stress control at shore fleet hospitals had to be improvised, and their suitability for Army reconditioning programs is questionable.

By G Day (the start of the ground war), the Navy had deployed makeshift combat stress centers forward to Marine medical battalion clearing and collection companies. An Army mental health officer with an Army armored brigade task force attached to a Marine division did coordinate for backup support from the Navy forward support medical company. The United Kingdom armored division had two forward psychiatric team (two officers and six enlisted each), one forward deployed. It is unclear whether these team could have been used to restore U.S. Army stress casualties had they come in contact/been required by circumstances, since the British use adhoc quartermaster elements as sites for their battle stress recovery units rather than collocating with medical treatment facilities.

There is a need to develop joint doctrine and training among U.S. Army, Air Force, and Navy mental health units. There is also a need to study how allied (multinational) combat stress control elements should cooperate, especially when individual elements cannot bring their entire medical support slices into the theater of operation. Joint doctrine planning with NATO allies would best take place in the context of the European Medical Psychiatry Working Group which meets annually but which often lacks U.S. participation.

SUMMARY OF CRITICAL ISSUES AND RECOMMENDATIONS

The organization, staffing, equipment, and training of mental health units deployed to the Gulf War were severely inadequate. Recently fielded combat stress control companies and detachments will be an improvement over the previous OM team concept. These new units need to operate according to doctrine, including their use in response to disaster and other humanitarian missions.

After action stress debriefings were important therapeutic interventions for units (and soldiers) exposed to extreme stress during the Gulf War. Unfortunately, only a limited number of mental health units/personnel were prepared to provide this service. Doctrine should require mental health intervention (stress debriefings) whenever a unit experiences extreme trauma (fatal training or operational accidents, terrorism, or combat exposure), and mental health personnel must be prepared for this mission.

The most effective Gulf War combat stress control efforts focused at brigade level. This should be the model for peacetime as well as wartime combat stress control operations. All deploying brigade size units (on a combat or a peacetime contingency mission) require organic mental health support.

Many division mental health personnel deployed to the Gulf War theater lacked credibility with battalion and brigade commanders (and their senior staff). Division mental health officers and behavioral science specialists (91Gs) need to be more senior and experienced. They must be competent soldiers and clinicians.

Units will always bring injured soldiers to the nearest hospital. Some hospitals did not have mental health personnel, and stress related casualties were inappropriately evacuated. All deployed hospitals require some mental health capability.

Battle fatigue treatment and disposition must focus on rapid return to duty in the soldier's original unit. The Gulf War evacuation policies and resources did not support this requirement.

CONCLUSION

What should we learn from mental health issues associated with the Gulf War? Based on the small number of soldiers evacuated from the Southwest Asia theater of operations for psychiatric reasons during the period August 1, 1990 to August 1, 1991, we obviously fielded a psychologically healthy Army. Taken together with other indicators of "problem behavior" (indiscipline, etc.) and our tremendously successful ground campaign, it is clear that Army active component combat forces deployed to the Gulf War were well trained and well led (according to our doctrine, these are two of the principal factors in preventing battle fatigue).

This war was not the challenge it could have been. Yet there were still soldiers exposed to the extreme stresses of war (inflicting and/or observing death, inflicting or being the victim of friendly fire, experiencing the horror of human remains, and encountering the victims of war—the men, women, and children killed, wounded, or made homeless). The Gulf War represents only one part of the spectrum of conflict. The Gulf War was the perfect American Army war because it fit our doctrine, our training, and our ground arsenal (Bolger, 1991). Our overwhelming success also helps ensure that the next war will be different—some other place on the spectrum of conflict with different problems requiring different solutions. Even so, the core of mental health issues associated with soldiers in combat will always be present. Only the range of issues and the magnitude of care required will change.

From a mental health perspective, the primary lesson we should derive from our Gulf War experience centers on preparation. Regardless of where on the spectrum of conflict we commit soldiers, war is traumatic, and mental health issues will always be important. Like other readiness issues, mental health resources need to be prepared today.

The mental health personnel deployed to the Gulf War theater were often not adequately trained as individuals or units, they were not well equipped, in many cases doctrine (for a variety of reasons) was not followed, and our efforts to deploy and use reserve component personnel and units were not successful. We were not ready. Our challenge is to develop and implement a peacetime mental health program that will allow us rapidly to transition to war. American soldiers deserve no less.

ACKNOWLEDGMENT

Headquarters, 7th Medical Command and the Walter Reed Army Institute of Research cosponsored an Operation Desert Shield & Storm lessons learned conference that provided the stimulus for this chapter. The document reflects the contributions of all conference participants.

APPENDIX

Conference Participants:

Captain Kelley Barham, U.S. Army, Research Consultant, HQ, 7th MEDCOM

Lieutenant Colonel John Bartz, U.S. Army, Department of Psychiatry, 97th General Hospital

Colonel Gregory Belenky, U.S. Army, Chief, Behavioral Biology Department, Walter Reed Army Institute of Research

Lieutenant Colonel Victor Bell, U.S. Army, Chief, Department of Psychiatry, 98th General Hospital

Major Richard Chance, U.S. Army, Division Psychiatrist, 8th ID

Captain Daniel Clark, U.S. Army, Psychologist, Division Mental Health, 3ID

Colonel William Cline, U.S. Army, Psychiatry Consultant, HQ 7th MEDCOM

Lieutenant Commander John Coogan, Senior Psychiatry Consultant, British Army of the Rhine

Major Kelley Cozza, U.S. Army, Division Psychiatrist, 3AD

Major William Evans, U.S. Army, Department of Psychiatry, 2nd General Hospital

Colonel Pilar Franco, U.S. Army, Department of Psychiatry, 97th General Hospital

Colonel Juan Garcia, U.S. Army, Corps Surgeon, HQ, V Corps

Major William Geeslin, U.S. Army, Social Work Services, 97th General Hospital

Captain Andrew Gergely, U.S. Army, Department of Psychiatry, 2nd General Hospital

Colonel Robert Griffin, U.S. Army, Corps Surgeon, HHC, VII Corps

Colonel Robert Griffin, U.S. Army Corps Surgeon, HHC, VII Corps

Colonel L. Steven Holsenbeck, U.S. Army, Department of Psychiatry, Eisenhower Army Medical Center, Ft. Gordon, GA
Shawnee Mission, KS

Colonel Albert Kopp, U.S. Army, Department of Psychiatry, 130th Station Hospital

Major Martin Leamon, U.S. Army, Department of Psychiatry, 97th General Hospital

Colonel F. J. Manning, U.S. Army, Director, Division of Neuropsychiatry, Walter Reed Army Institute of Research, Washington, DC

Lieutenant Colonel Marrero, U.S. Army, USAF, 86th Medical Group

Colonel James Martin, U.S. Army, Medical Research Unit-Europe, HQ, 7th MEDCOM

Major Dorothy O'Keefe, U.S. Army, Chief, Department of Psychiatry, 2nd General Hospital

Lieutenant Colonel Marylyn Schneider, U.S. Army, Department of Psychiatry, 130th Station Hospital

Lieutenant Colonel Ross Shuman, U.S. Army, Department of Psychiatry, 98th General Hospital

Captain Gary Southwell, U.S. Army, Division Psychologist, 30th Field Hospital

Major Loree Sutton, U.S. Army, HHC, 1st Armored Division

Captain Robert Waterman, U.S. Army, Division Psychiatrist, 3AD

REFERENCES

Bolger, D. (1991). "The ghosts of Omdurman." *Parameters*, XXI(3):28–39.
Levens, L. and B. Schemmer. (1991). "An exclusive interview with General Gordon Sullivan." *Armed Forces J. International*, October, 54–58.

16

The Future Practice of Combat Psychiatry

Gregory Belenky and James A. Martin

INTRODUCTION

From our experiences during the Gulf War (described in Chapter 7, this volume), we have developed guidelines for the conduct of mental health operations in future conflicts. These guidelines apply to large scale air land battle combat operations, to smaller scale combat operations, and to military operations other than war, including peacekeeping and humanitarian missions. We offer them as suggestions and considerations for the planning and conduct of mental health operations. The conduct of such operations requires flexibility, adaptability, and improvisation. In the past, operational mental health guidelines have, often with best intentions, been reduced to and presented as a simplistic formula to be rigidly applied. The complexities surrounding the prevention and treatment of stress casualties cannot be covered in a few phrases capped off by an acronym. The means and techniques of conducting mental health operations are presently evolving rapidly as both the tactical decentralization of the theater of operations increases and improvements in telecommunications extend the reach of mental health teams and increase their integration into combat operations. The collection and analysis of detailed psychosocial and psychophysiological information from individual soldiers and units done up to this point for after the fact research purposes is becoming a real time enterprise. These data and their analyses are being made available to command for the purpose of operational planning and to both command and mental health personnel to guide individual and organizational interventions and thus to increase individual and unit effectiveness and decrease stress casualties.

Mental health operations entail both preventing and treating combat and operational stress casualties. With respect to prevention, factors that enhance individual and unit combat effectiveness can decrease combat stress casualties. Conversely, factors that reduce individual and unit combat effectiveness can increase combat stress casualties.   These factors include battle intensity and type, leadership and cohesion, combat experience, training and fitness, hydration, sleep and food, personal situation, personal qualities, and ethical climate within the unit (Grinker and Speigel, 1943; Mullins and Glass, 1973; Belenky 1987; Belenky, Noy, and Solomon 1987).   Favorable weightings of these factors reduce stress casualties and increase effectiveness. The prevention of these casualties is a command responsibility most effectively met by the combined and coordinated efforts of line and mental health personnel.

Acute combat stress casualties are typically referred to medical or mental health personnel by the soldier's immediate chain of command. Treatment is most effective if rapid, brief, in or near the unit, and conducted with the involvement of soldiers from the unit when that is possible. Treatment itself consists of physical replenishment (water, food, sleep) and a chance to tell one's story to a comprehending and sympathetic person or persons. The chance to tell one's story is, in effect, a post combat debriefing/event reconstruction. It is best done in situ, in the unit, in groups, as a general preventive measure, without identifying or singling out as a patient the soldier who was referred. For a case example of this technique, see Chapter 7.

In contemporary combat operations, units are dispersed and maneuver over a large area. In military operations other than war, units are more fixed in location but again dispersed over a large area. Operational units coordinate their actions through a combination of satellite based navigation and local and satellite based radio frequency communication. Mental health work requires face to face contact with soldiers preferably in situ in their unit. Mental health personnel should be deployed at the level of, or be able to reach easily, the operational unit of maneuver. The operational unit of maneuver (in the U.S. Army, the battalion) is the highest unit of shared experience.

ORGANIZING FOR THE MISSION

Mental health personnel should be organized into three person teams, consisting of two officers and one noncommissioned officer. The two officers can be any combination of psychiatrist, psychologist, and social worker. The noncommissioned officer should be a medical or behavioral science specialist. Each team should be able to move, navigate, and communicate. This requires an all terrain vehicle (HUMMV or equivalent), a global positioning system receiver (GPS), maps, and a radio. In the not too distant future, the GPS, maps, and radio will be integrated into the soldier computer, carried by and effectively linking all soldiers, independent of rank, position, or echelon of command and control.

In combat operations, one mental health team should be deployed with each maneuver brigade and attached to the medical company in the brigade's support battalion. A brigade typically consists of 2000 to 3000 soldiers divided into to three to four maneuver battalions and one support battalion. A brigade is small enough and compact enough to be served by a mobile, three person mental health team. The team will do most of its work at the company, platoon, and squad/crew level. Deploying with a brigade gives the team practical access to battalions, companies, platoons, and squads/crews. Battles are won or lost at the battalion, company, and platoon, squad/crew level (Marshall, 1978; English, 1984). The squad/crew level is effectively the smallest unit of shared experience, the repository of powerful primary group ties, and the focus of mental health and, for that matter, command intervention.

Laying the Groundwork for Effective Operations

Once attached to the medical company of a brigade, the mental health team should lay the groundwork for effective operation. The team should introduce itself with a brief statement of purpose to the entire operational chain of command, working down from the brigade commander and brigade staff through battalion, company, platoon, and squad/crew. At the platoon and squad/crew level, the team should carry out its introductions, walking from tank to tank and fighting vehicle to fighting vehicle. At all levels of command and control, the team should introduce itself with something like, "We are your mental health team. We are attached to the medical company. We will be available during the upcoming operations to talk with anyone who wishes to talk to us. After engagements, we will come by to do systematic debriefings and battle reconstructions. It would help us if you would tell us what you expect the upcoming operations will be like." The medical system and the chaplaincy are alternate lines of command and information flow, paralleling the operational one. The team should introduce itself to the brigade and battalion chaplains and to the brigade, battalion, and company medical personnel.

Over the course of the introductions, the team should be assessing the organizational climate, level of stress and adaptation, morale, and psychological preparation and readiness for combat or mission performance of the maneuver units. Also, the team should be collecting and collating information to construct the anticipated shape of the impending operation as seen through the eyes of personnel from brigade headquarters down to crew and squad. The team will then be able to follow the course of the battle, note where the operation deviates from expectation, competently debrief and treat stress casualties during the operation, and, after the operation, identify specific units and events as high priority foci for post combat debriefings/battle reconstructions.

The work of a mental health team is approximately one third prevention and consultation, one third treatment of acute stress casualties, and one third after-action debriefings and event reconstructions combined with further command consultation. This distribution of work is depicted in Figure 16.1. In the Gulf War, we observed that the bulk of the medical assets, including mental health personnel, packed up to go home immediately after the cease-fire. This was appropriate for medical and surgical personnel, but inappropriate for mental health personnel. The work of the mental health teams was at that point only one half to two thirds completed.

Figure 16.1
Mental Health Team Work Load by Task in Relation to a Five-Day Battle

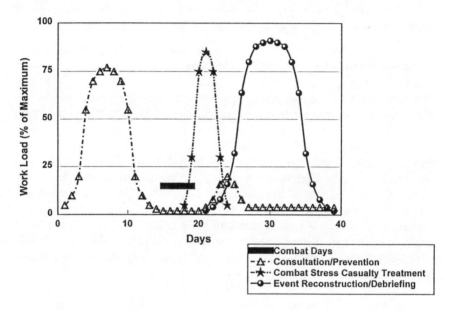

Command Consultation and Casualty Prevention

Combat leaders in the U.S. Army are well informed and sophisticated in their approach to issues of morale, leadership, cohesion, and combat effectiveness. They welcome well informed advice and consultation from mental health personnel. This is especially true if mental health personnel are knowledgeable and couch their advice in terms of improving operational effectiveness. Command and mental health personnel work on common ground, making possible mutually supportive action. Medical monitoring and computer modeling, already extensively used in preventive medicine and in the prediction of physical casualties, are being extended and applied to the psychophysiologi-cal areas of sleep and performance and to the socio-psychological areas of morale, cohesion, and unit climate. Using these results, both commanders and mental health personnel can make effective individual and organizational interventions. Psychophysiological monitoring will include means to measure sleep under operational conditions, models to predict performance on the basis of prior sleep, and on-line real-time monitoring of alertness and performance. Sociopsychological monitoring, presently used in deployed U.S. forces, will include tools to measure in real time individual and unit well being, morale, and cohesion.

Treatment of Acute Combat Stress Casualties

Acute combat and operational stress casualties are those casualties emerging during or immediately after combat. These casualties develop in and around areas where physical and mental trauma have been the greatest. Their arrival at the battalion aid station tends to lag the physical casualties by a day or two. Acute stress casualties almost invariably show signs of both mental and physical stress. They are typically survivors of some intense battle or other demoralizing, life threatening event. The treatment is as much physical as mental, with the focus being on physical replenishment, reversal of demoralization, and restoration of personal morale and mental equilibrium. In practical terms, this means providing the soldier with water and food, sleep, and a chance to tell his or her story to a comprehending and sympathetic ear. This latter can be on an individual basis with mental health personnel or in groups as an event debriefing/reconstruction. Such treatment should be as far forward as possible (e.g., at the battalion aid station or in situ in the unit). The critical element in the treatment of an acute stress casualty is the restoration of the interpersonal bonds between the soldier and his or her comrades. The treatment is not complete without this restoration. The individual physical replenishment, reversal of demoralization, and restoration of morale and personal equilibrium are to bring the soldier to a mental and physical state where he or she is capable of making this reintegration. Successful treatment is defined operationally as a return of the soldier to effective duty with his or her unit.

Pharmacotherapy in the Treatment of Acute Combat Stress Casualties

There is no conclusive evidence that any pharmacotherapeutic agent is of benefit in the treatment of acute combat stress reactions or the prevention of posttraumatic stress disorder (PTSD). In the Vietnam War, neuroleptics, benzodiazepines, and the then available antidepressants were used but to no documented effect. Currently, the U.S. Army leaves the decision regarding the use of psychotropic agents in the hands of the treating physician.

The neuroleptics, also called major tranquilizers (e.g., chlorpromazine [Thorazine®]), are used to treat psychotic conditions such as schizophrenia or mania. The benzodiazepines, also called minor tranquilizers (e.g., diazepam

[Valium®]), are used to relieve anxiety and promote sleep. The tricyclic antidepressants (e.g., imipramine [Tofranil®]) and related compounds are used to treat depression. A new class of antidepressants, the selective serotonin reuptake inhibitors (SSRIs) (e.g., fluoxetine [Prozac®]), have been developed since the Vietnam War and have not been used to treat combat stress reactions or prevent PTSD.

It is our view that neuroleptics and benzodiazepines have no role in the treatment of combat stress casualties or the prevention of PTSD. Anecdotal observations by the Israeli Defense Force during the 1973 Arab–Israeli War and the 1982 War in Lebanon suggest that the use of neuroleptics and benzodiazepines, while effective in symptom reduction over the first few hours, interferes with coping and readjustment, further debilitating the soldier, reducing the likelihood of full recovery over the two to three days post-trauma, and creating longer-term disability. It is also our impression that mental health professionals in the Gulf War were poised to use benzodiazepines liberally had there been large numbers of combat stress casualties. Benzodiazepines are effective in reducing anxiety and promoting sleep. It is questionable whether pharmacologic relief from anxiety and pharmacologic sleep induction are needed for acute combat stress casualties. The simple fact of rearward evacuation relieves anxiety. This, combined with the fact that most combat stress casualties are sleep deprived, is sufficient to promote sleep. That mental health personnel in the Gulf War were eager to administer benzodiazepines reflects their belief that these agents were therapeutically indicated and that combat stress casualties would be unmanageable if not sedated. Both beliefs are unfounded.

The SSRIs may have a beneficial effect in treating combat stress casualties, especially if combined with event reconstruction and debriefing. These agents are, relative to older antidepressants, free from side effects, including performance impairment. They have, to our knowledge, not been tried in the management of acute combat stress reaction or the prevention of posttraumatic stress disorder. These agents appear in clinical settings to improve day to day performance and increase resiliency in depressed, demoralized individuals. We would recommend prospective, randomized, double blind studies of their efficacy when used immediately posttrauma in all individuals exposed to the trauma whether they are at that point symptomatic or not. Other agents may prove effective in reducing the risk of an acute stress reaction progressing to chronic PTSD. What is necessary in our view is controlled, prospective studies upon which to base recommendations for clinical practice.

Postcombat Debriefing and Event Reconstruction

Postcombat event reconstructions and debriefings come in a variety of closely related forms with substantial overlap in methods and goals. Post combat event reconstructions and debriefings range from the command conducted operational debriefing of a combat unit focused on the accurate reconstruction of a complex event or events to a mental health personnel conducted clinical debriefing of an individual or small group focused on emotional release and reversing demoralization. The operational debriefing was first fully developed as a historical tool by S. L. A. Marshall during World War II (Marshall, 1978). Marshall found that by assembling a combat unit soon after a firefight, setting rank aside and making all personnel equal witnesses, and encouraging all to contribute, he could develop a detailed, coherent account of an action. This type of debriefing not only served to reconstruct the battle, but produced valuable operational lessons and served to reintegrate and restore morale in the unit following a difficult action. Clinical debriefings grew out of clinical work with individuals and groups and have developed into the critical incident stress debriefing (CISD). CISDs are carried out routinely for civilian police, fire, rescue, and emergency medical personnel following a traumatic event. There is a large area of overlap between the two. Operational debriefings lead to improvement in the individual and unit Well Being in the units debriefed; clinical debriefings can generate valuable operational lessons. Overall, the techniques used in operational and clinical debriefings are similar; the intent of one is the complement of the intent of the other.

The bulk of the physical casualties will be treated during or immediately after combat. The bulk of debriefing and event reconstruction will be done after combat. Thus, medical personnel will be available to supplement the mental health teams in after-action debriefings and event reconstructions. As this work requires the time and the willingness to do it rather than any specific training or expertise, these non mental-health medical personnel can be useful in carrying out a program of systematic debriefing at the squad/crew, platoon, or company level for all those involved in combat operations. With regard to other resources, it is our impression that many chaplains are convinced of the usefulness of debriefings and event reconstructions and are already well informed regarding the techniques involved. They are the natural partners of mental health personnel and other medical personnel in this work. Finally, commanders will often make the time to participate in debriefings and event reconstructions in units under their command.

Mental Health Operations and the Revolution in Military Affairs

The rapid digitization of the battlefield and the integration of networked computers into military operations is creating what has been termed a revolution in military affairs. At the most basic and universal level, the U.S. Army plans to equip each soldier with a computer. This device will be worn as part of the basic combat load and will include the functional capacity of a personal computer, the software and hardware to interface with GPS, the software and hardware for secure voice and data transmission through local area radio frequency computer networking and satellite up-and-down links, and helmet mounted display of topographical and other relevant information. Incorporated will be personnel status monitoring (PSM) hardware and software. This would include a suite of sensors to measure a variety of biomedical parameters. In addition to pulse, temperature, and state of hydration, this projected suite will unobtrusively monitor sleep, alertness, and performance. Further, the PSM will contain tools to assess individual psychological status and unit organizational climate in real time. All of this information will be available to command for use in operational planning and to medical and mental health personnel for conducting mental health operations. This will allow the intelligent management of sleep to optimize performance by the designated unit sleep manager. It will support group-level interventions by both command and mental health personnel to improve individual and unit morale, cohesion, and effectiveness. These data will be available at all levels of command and control. These data available from soldiers through their networked computers will be independent of their medical records. Soldiers' medical records are and will remain confidential. Present plans envisage soldiers carrying their medical records encrypted on a microchip embedded in a dog tag. This dog tag will be physically separate from the soldier's computer and the soldier's medical records stored on the dog tag will be accessible only by medical personnel possessing the appropriate decryption key.

A recent example of the acquisition, analysis, and feedback to command of unit organizational and climate data occurred in Operation Uphold Democracy in Haiti. A human dimensions research team (HDRT) was deployed from the Walter Reed Army Institute of Research in support of Operation Uphold Democracy (Halverson et al., 1995). This team collected detailed questionnaire data from over one third of the 11,000+ American soldiers in Haiti. The team analyzed the data and was able to feed back to commanders the general well being, morale, and other psychosocial data on over 100 companies within seven days of completing data collection.

In the future, such data will be collected as often as needed from soldiers through the soldier computer and analyzed as collected. Feedback to command and to mental health personnel will be in real time. Mental health personnel will use these data and their own observations in consultation to command. Command will use these data in operational planning and in developing interventions. Mental health personnel will use data from battalions, companies, and smaller units to estimate the climate and atmosphere in the units from which they are getting referrals. These data will give mental health personnel a clearer picture as to whether a given soldier's difficulties are effectively his or her own, or the tip of the iceberg of a dysfunctional unit. This will, in turn, lead to more effective individual and, where appropriate, group intervention and provide further substance for command consultation. Increasingly, mental health operations will be integrated into the conduct of operations in general. For the current status of work in this area, see the Division of Neuropsychiatry, Walter Reed Army Institute of Research, Home Page on the World Wide Web at (http://wrair-www.army.mil/np/nphp.htm).

SUMMARY

This then is our picture of mental health teams in future operations: The teams will be small, multidisciplinary, and mobile and support operational units of brigade size. They will have at their disposal a wealth of psychophysiological and psychosocial data, collected from soldiers through the soldier computer and analyzed in real time. In support of this data collection and analysis, the teams will carry computers, radio frequency linked for voice, video, and data to each other and to relevant command and control elements. These data will be available to and used by commanders in operational planning (e.g., effective sleep management to optimize individual and unit performance) and will be used by the mental health teams in command consultation and in individual and group interventions. Mental health teams will deploy to a theater of operations early in the course of the operation and leave at the end. Event reconstructions and debriefings will be a large part of the work of the mental health teams. These reconstructions and debriefings will be conducted after the battle or battles, after the cease-fire, after the cusp of the operation.

At the heart of the mental health teams' work will be face to face contact with individual soldiers and small units as well as elements in their chain of command. Depending on the degree of decentralization and the fluidity of the battlefield, this could be done remotely through video teleconference links. These face to face contacts will be for the purpose of initially laying the groundwork for and later conducting post combat debriefing and event reconstruction and treating and rapidly reintegrating acute stress casualties back into their units.

The operations of the mental health teams will be integrated with line operations to an unprecedented degree, with an iterative/recursive interaction with command, unit, and individual in the form of face-to-face interviewing and debriefings and more objective assessment of psychophysiological and psychosocial variables. The actual work of the mental health teams in an operational setting will be quite different from, and extend far beyond, traditional mental health work in an outpatient clinic or inpatient ward. To be effective, team members must be experts in operational mental health, knowledgeable about the conduct of combat operations, and facile in the use of and limitations of the technical (data gathering, analysis, and communication) tools at their disposal.

REFERENCES

Belenky, G., S. Noy, and Z. Solomon. (1987). "Battle stress, morale, cohesion, combat effectiveness, heroism, and psychiatric casualties: The Israeli experience." In G. Belenky (ed.), *Contemporary Studies in Combat Psychiatry*. Westport, Conn.: Greenwood, 11–20.

Belenky, G. (1987). "Varieties of reaction & adaptation to combat experience." Bull. *Menninger Clinic*, 51:64–79.

English, J. (1984). *On Infantry*. New York: Praeger.

Grinker, R. R. and J. P Spiegel. (1943). *Men under Stress*. New York: McGraw Hill.

Halverson, R.R., P.D. Bliese, R.E. Moore, and C.A. Castro. (1995). *Psychological Well-Being and Physical Health Symptoms of Soldiers Deployed for Operation Uphold Democracy: A Summary of Human Dimensions Research in Haiti*. Defense Technical Information Center Report, DTIC ADA 298125.

Marshall, S. L. A. (1978). *Men Against Fire*. Gloucester, Mass.: Peter Smith Press.

Mullins, W. S. and A. J. Glass. (eds.) (1973). *Neuropsychiatry in World War II. Vol. II. Overseas Theaters*. Washington, D.C.: Office of the Surg Gen, Dept. of the Army.

Simpkin, R. (1985). *Race to the Swift: Thoughts on 21st Century Warfare*. London: Brassey's Defense Publishers.

Further Readings

Bartemeier, L. H., L. S. Kubie, K. A. Menninger, J. Romano and J. D. Whitehorn. (1946). "Combat exhaustion." *J. Nerv. and Mental Dis.*, 104:358–389.

Belenky, G. L. (1987). "Varieties of reaction and adaptation to combat experience." *Bull. Menninger Clinic*, 51:64–79.

Belenky, G. (ed.) (1987). *Contemporary Studies in Combat Psychiatry*. Westport, Conn.: Greenwood.

Bourne, P. G. (1970). "Military psychiatry and the Vietnam experience." *Amer. J. Psychiatry*, 127:123–130.

Camp, N. M. (1993). "The Vietnam war and the ethics of combat psychiatry." *Amer. J. Psychiatry*, 150:1000–1010.

Copp, T. and B. McAndrew. (1990). *Battle Exhaustion: Soldiers and Psychiatrists in the Canadian Army, 1939–1945*. Montreal: McGill Queen's University Press.

Figley, C. R. (ed.) (1985). *Trauma and Its Wake: Study and Treatment of Post Traumatic Stress Disorder*. New York: Brunner/Mazel.

Gal, R. and A. D. Mangelsdorff. (eds.) (1991). *Handbook of Military Psychology*. West Sussex, England: John Wiley & Sons.

Glass, A. J. (1953). "Preventive psychiatry in the combat zone." *U.S. Armed Forces Med. J.*, 4:683–692.

Glass, A. J. (ed.) (1973). *Neuropsychiatry in World War II, Vol. II, Overseas Theaters*. Washington, D.C.: Office of the Surgeon General, Department of the Army.

Glass, A. J. and R. J. Bernucci. (eds.) (1966). *Neuropsychiatry in World War II, Vol. I, Zone of the Interior*. Washington, D.C.: Office of the Surgeon General, Department of the Army.

Grinker, R. R. and Spiegel, J.P. (1963). *Men Under Stress*. New York: McGraw Hill.

Hendin, H. and A. P. Haas. (1984). Wounds of War: *The Psychological Aftermath of Combat in Vietnam*. New York: Basic Books.

Holmes, R. (1985). *Acts of War: The Behavior of Men in Battle*. New York: The Free Press.

Jones, F. D. (1982). "Combat stress: Tripartite model." *Int. Rev. Army, Navy, and Air Force Med. Serv.*, 55:247–254.

Jones, F. D., L. R. Sparacino, V. L. Wilcox and J. M. Rothberg. (eds.) (1994)."Military psychiatry: Preparing in peace for war." In *Textbook of Military Medicine*. Washington, D.C.: Office of the Surgeon General of the Army and The Borden Institute.

Jones, F.D., L. R. Sparacino, V. L. Wilcox, J. M. Rothberg and J. W. Stokes. (eds.) (1995). "War psychiatry." In *Textbook of Military Medicine*. Washington, D.C.: Office of the Surgeon General of the Army and The Borden Institute.

Keegen, J. (1978). *The Face of Battle*. New York: Penguin Books.

Kellett, A. (1982). *Combat Motivation: The Behavior of Soldiers in Battle*. Boston: Kluwer Nijhoff.

Levav, I., H. Greenfield and E. Baruch. (1979). "Psychiatric combat reactions during the Yom Kippur War." *Amer. J. Psychiatry*, 136:637–641.

Menninger, W. C. (1948). *Psychiatry in a Troubled World: Yesterday's War and Today's Challenges*. New York: Macmillan.

Rahe, R. H. (1988). "Acute versus chronic psychological reactions to combat." *Mil. Med.*, 153:365–372.

Ranson, S. W. (1949). "The normal battle reaction: Its relation to pathologic battle reaction. Combat psychiatry." Bull. U.S. Army Med. Dep., 9:3–11.

Renner, J. A., Jr. (1973). "The changing patterns of psychiatric problems in Vietnam." *Comp. Psychiatry*, 14:169–181.

Salmon, T. W. and N. Fenton. (1929). *Neuropsychiatry in the American Expeditionary Forces*. Vol. X. Washington, D.C.: USGPO.

Shalit, B. (1988). *The Psychology of Conflict and Combat*. New York: Praeger.

Shay, J. (1994). *Achilles in Vietnam: Combat Trauma and the Undoing of Character*. New York: Atheneum.

Sobel, R. (1947). "The 'old sergeant' syndrome." *Psychiatry*, 10:315–321.

Soloman, Z. (1993). *Combat Stress Reaction: The Enduring Tool of War*. New York: Plenum Press.

Sonnenberg, S. M., A. S. Bland and J. A. Talbott. (eds.) (1985). *The Trauma of War: Stress and Recovery in Vietnam Veterans*. Washington, D.C.: American Psychiatric Association.

Steiner, M. and M. Neumann. (1978). "Traumatic neurosis and social support in the Yom Kippur War returnees." *Mil. Med.*, 12:866–868.

Stouffer, S. A. et al. (1949). *Studies in Social Psychology in World War II. Vol. 2. The American Soldier: Combat and Its Aftermath*. Princeton, N.J.: Princeton University Press.

Swank, R. L. and W. E. Marchand. (1946). "Combat neuroses." *Archives of Neurol.*, 55:236–246.

Yerkes, S. A. (1993). "The 'un comfort able': Making sense of adaptation in a war zone." *Mil. Med.*, 158:421–423.

Index

About the Editors and Contributors

Paul T. Bartone, Ph.D., Major, U.S. Army Medical Service Corps, is currently the Commander of the U.S. Army Medical Research Unit-Europe in Heidelberg, Germany. Major Bartone is a research psychologist.

Gregory Belenky, M.D., Colonel, U.S. Army Medical Corps, is currently the Director of the Division of Neuropsychiatry at the Walter Reed Army Institute of Research in Washington, DC. Colonel Belenky served as a mental health officer in the 2nd Armored Cavalry Regiment.

Spencer J. Campbell, Major, U.S. Army Medical Service Corps, is currently an instructor in the Behavioral Science Division of the Army Medical Center and School at Fort Sam Houston, Texas. Major Campbell served as a social worker in the First Cavalry Division.

Daniel W. Clark, Ph.D., is a former Captain in the U.S. Army. He is employed by the Washington State Police. Mr. Clarke served as a clinical psychologist in the 1st Armored Division.

William R. Cline, M.D., Colonel (Ret.), U.S. Medical Corps, lives in Washington, DC. He was the Neuropsychiatry Consultant of Headquarters, 7th Medical Command in Germany during the Persian Gulf War.

Michael P. Dinneen, M.D., Lieutenant Commander, U.S. Navy Medical Corps, is assigned to the U.S. Navy Medical Center in Bethesda, MD. Commander Dinneen served as a psychiatrist on the *U.S.S. Comfort*.

Charles C. Engel, Jr., Major, U. S. Army (Reserves) Medical Service Corps, is an assistant instructor at the University of Washington in Seattle, WA. Major Engel served as a clinical psychologist in the 1st Cavalry Division.

Joe G. Fagan, M.D., Colonel (Ret.), U.S. Army Medical Corps, was the Army Theater Psychiatry Consultant in the Persian Gulf War. He previously served as the Neurology and Psychiatry Consultant to the Surgeon General of the U.S. Army. Colonel Fagan is a psychiatrist.

Robert K. Gifford, Ph.D., Colonel, U.S. Army, Medical Service Corps, presently is the Chief of the Department of Military Psychiatry at the Walter Reed Army Institute of Research in Washington, DC. Colonel Gifford is a research psychologist.

Deborah Hickey, Colonel, U.S. Army currently serves on the staff of Madigan Army Medical Center, Fort Lewis, WA. Colonel Hickey served as an OM Team psychiatrist.

L. Stephen Holsenbeck, M.D., Colonel (Ret.), U. S. Army Medical Corps, currently resides in Colorado. Colonel Holsenbeck was an OM Team Commander during the Gulf War.

Joyce C. Humphrey, Colonel, U.S. Army (Reserves) Nurse Corps, is a professor at the University of Massachusetts. Colonel Humphrey is a psychiatric nurse. She served as a senior headquarters staff officer during the Gulf War.

Robert T. Joy, M.D., Colonel (Ret.), U.S. Army Medical Corps, is the Chair of the Department of Military History at the Uniformed Services University of Health Sciences in Bethesda, Maryland.

Faris R. Kirkland, Ph.D., Lieutenant Colonel (Ret.), U.S. Army Field Artillery Corps, was a battalion commander in Vietnam. He is a military historian who has written extensively on combat and its historical context.

Mary Laedtke, Major, U.S. Army Medical Service Corps, is an occupational therapist at Eisenhower Army Medical Center in Georgia. Major Laedtke was an OM Team member during the Gulf War.

Scott C. Marcy, Colonel, U.S. Army Armor Corps, is a Pentagon staff officer. He was a squadron commander in the 2nd Armored Cavalry Regiment during the Gulf War.

David H. Marlowe, Ph.D., is a Senior Scientist at the Department of Military Psychiatry at the Walter Reed Army Institute of Research in Washington, DC. Dr. Marlowe was the previous Chief of the Department of Military Psychiatry at the Walter Reed Army Institute of Research.   Dr. Marlowe is a social anthropologist.

James A. Martin, Ph.D., Colonel (Ret.), is an Associate Professor, Bryn Mawr College Graduate School of Social Work and Social Research, Bryn Mawr College, Bryn Mawr, PA.   Colonel Martin served as a mental health officer in the 2nd Armored Cavalry Regiment during the Gulf War.

James Pecano, Ph.D., Major, U.S. Army (Reserves) Medical Service Corps, is a clinical psychologist in Pleasantown, California.   Major Pecano served as an OM Team psychologist during the Gulf War.

Paul W. Ragan, M.D., Commander, U.S. Navy Medical Corps, is assigned to the Navy Outpatient Psychiatry Service at the National Institute of Health, Bethesda, Maryland.   Commander Ragan served as a psychiatrist in support of the 2nd Marine Expeditionary Force.

David C. Ruck, M.D., is a former Lieutenant Colonel in the U.S. Army Medical Corps. He is in private practice in Georgia. Dr. Ruck served as an OM Team psychiatrist.

Linette R. Sparacino, M.A., is a Medical Editor at the Borden Institute in the Office of the Surgeon General of the Army, Washington DC. Ms. Sparacino edited *Military Psychiatry*, *Preparing in Peace for War*, and *War Psychiatry*.

James W. Stokes, M.D., Colonel, U.S. Army Medical Corps, is the Chief of the Psychiatry and Neurology Branch at the Army Medical Department and School in Fort Sam Houston, Texas. Colonel Stokes is a psychiatrist.

Loree Sutton, M.D., Lieutenant Colonel, U.S. Army Medical Corps, is a student at the Army Command and General Staff College, Leavenworth, KS. Colonel Sutton served as a psychiatrist in the 1st Armored Division.

Kathleen M. Wright, Ph.D., is the Deputy Chief for Research in the Department of Military Psychiatry at the Walter Reed Army Institute of Research in Washington, DC. Dr. Wright is a clinical psychologist who specialized in traumatic events. She was one of the few civilian women allowed into the combat arena during the Gulf War.

ISBN 0-275-95631-8

HARDCOVER BAR CODE